NG TEAM ORGANIZATION AND FUNCTIONING

Results of a Study of the
DIVISION OF NURSING EDUCATION
Teachers College, Columbia University

ELEANOR C. LAMBERTSEN, R.N., A.M.
Instructor in Nursing Education

Published for the
DIVISION OF NURSING EDUCATION
TEACHERS COLLEGE PRESS
TEACHERS COLLEGE • COLUMBIA UNIVERSITY
NEW YORK

Printed in the United States of America

FOREWORD

THIS PUBLICATION is the outgrowth of experimentation designed to solve the problem of utilizing nursing personnel in hospitals most advantageously.

Much has been said and written about the critical shortage of nursing personnel, about the plight of hospitals that are insufficiently staffed, and about the personal problems of the patient who needs professional nursing care which is unobtainable. The factors which have contributed to this increasingly serious situation are extremely complex, and no simple solution seems possible. There is, however, no justification for postponing all-out and unremitting attack on the problem.

In its report, "Program for the Nursing Profession," published in 1948, the Committee on Function of Nursing appointed by the Division of Nursing Education of Teachers College recommended several types of research that should be undertaken. The approach, the Committee cautioned, should be away from current practice and analysis of present activities and toward more venturesome experimentation to establish new standards for future practice. Experimentation in nursing is difficult to initiate because of the inevitable resistance to change and the understandable fear of failure. However, the Committee's clear mandate to take the next step without delay led the staff of the Division of Nursing Education to start planning for experimentation.

When financial support from other sources could not be procured, sufficient money to get started was released from the Teachers College general funds. A blueprint was prepared for a broad and long-term study of the function of nursing. At the same time, related and more highly specialized studies and experimentation were planned. Hypotheses about the scope and nature of the function of nursing were set up for testing. A plan for organizing hospital nursing staffs to achieve patient-centered care was designed, based upon utilization of all nursing personnel in the interest of economy and efficiency.

Experimentation was initiated on a limited scale under Amelia Leino in Morrisania Hospital and the Woman's Hospital. Subsequently, when funds for research and for nursing service administration were made available by the W. K. Kellogg Foundation, the study was expanded under the direction of Miss Eleanor Lambertsen. With the cooperation of Commissioner Kogel of the Department of Hospitals, New York City, the nursing staff of that department and the Teachers College Nursing Education Division research staff developed and put into effect at the new Delafield Hospital a plan for organizing nursing service from the start on a team basis.

As experimentation has progressed, changes in the concept have evolved; and as group after group of graduate nurses has tested them in practice, the principles have been clarified. In this publication these tentatively held concepts and principles and the general plan of the organization and functioning of teams are described. The discussion should help remove current confusion among many hospital administrators, doctors, and nurses regarding what constitutes a nursing team. Merely assigning professional nurses, practical nurses, nurse's aides, and student nurses to work in the same ward unit does not necessarily make a team. Unless the workers or players are united for a common purpose, unless they know the roles they are expected to play and are all familiar with the rules, unless they know the signals and willingly accept and follow the leadership of the team captain, there can be no team.

It is maintained in this book that the nursing team, comprised as it is of personnel with different functions and types of preparation, is able to achieve for a group of patients a quality of nursing care that would be unattainable by the same workers when assigned to fragmented tasks and individual procedures. The author does not claim that a final answer to the question of team organization and functioning has been reached or that proof is available that organizing nursing service administration on a team basis is the most effective and economical method possible. There is considerable evidence, however, that all nursing service personnel derive more satisfaction from their work when functioning as team members.

As the experiment goes forward, additional steps should be taken to study other aspects of nursing service administration, such as the ratio of professional nurses to nonprofessional personnel, and the differentiation of hospital and institutional service from nursing service. The theories and principles presented herewith for wider consideration are fundamental to further experimentation in economically providing an improved quality of individualized patient care in hospitals.

R. LOUISE MCMANUS
Professor of Nursing Education
Teachers College, Columbia University

CONTENTS

1. INTRODUCTION

EXPERIMENTATION and research in the organization and functioning of nursing teams were initiated by the Division of Nursing Education of Teachers College, Columbia University in December, 1949. At that time, the Morrisania Hospital, associated with the Department of Hospitals of New York City, made available two of its wards as research units. In July, 1950, The Woman's Hospital, a voluntary hospital which also is in New York City, agreed to participate in the study.

The purpose of the study was to find the best means by which to organize hospital nursing service personnel so as to achieve the most effective patient-centered nursing care. (36:1) *

This initial phase of the study was conducted in separate ward units of the two cooperating hospitals where the philosophy and over-all methodology of initiating the nursing team were developed, and factors were identified which influenced effective functioning of the nursing team. It became obvious that the ward was too small a base for experimentation; that it was necessary to include the entire nursing service of the hospital.

The Division of Nursing Education of Teachers College took the next logical step, seeking a hospital willing to cooperate in the organization, on a team basis, of an entire nursing service department. The Department of Hospitals of the City of New York expressed a willingness to cooperate on this larger scale.

On August 1, 1950, financial support for the continuation of the study was provided through a grant to the Division of Nursing Education by the W. K. Kellogg Foundation, Battle Creek, Michigan. The grant was for a period of five years, and covered research in nursing service administration, including the study of nursing team organization and functioning.

That phase of the research which is concerned with the study of the nursing team is entitled Project I, and reads in part as follows:

To set up an educational program in nursing service administration in a demonstration teaching center in one or more hospitals in New York

* The first number in parentheses refers to item in the Bibliography (pp. 77 to 80); the second number, to pages within the reference.

City, where students enrolled in Teachers College, Division of Nursing Education, may have the following laboratory experiences in field work courses that would then be organized as an integral part of the program preparing them for nursing service administrative positions:

1. Concurrent observation and practice of general nursing service administration for students preparing for positions as:

(a) Director of Nursing, in charge of a nursing service department.

(b) Assistant Nursing Service Administrator, in charge of the personnel program, the on-the-job training program, or a clinical division or unit.

2. Concurrent practice as staff nurses in a nursing service organized on a team basis for nurses in the prespecialization program.

3. Internship program in nursing service administration for nurses who have completed their program of organized study and who need closer observation of and supervised experience in performing the functions of directors of nursing service and assistant directors.

4. Concurrent participation in action research related to the direct improvement of bedside nursing care of patients in the demonstration hospitals.

Upon receipt of the grant, the proposals of Project I were presented to the Department of Hospitals, with the result that the facilities of a new hospital, The Francis Delafield, were made available for study.

Delafield Hospital is unique in at least two respects. First, it is owned and operated by the City of New York, Department of Hospitals, although its medical care program is provided and directed by the Columbia-Presbyterian Medical Center Board, and appointments to the medical staff are recommended by that Board and approved by the Department of Hospitals. Second, it is a special hospital for treatment and research in the care of patients with cancer and allied diseases.

On October 31, 1950, a conference was called at Delafield by the Director of Nursing Education and Nursing Service of the Department of Hospitals, at the direction of the Commissioner of Hospitals, Department of Hospitals. At this conference, plans were discussed for nursing and nursing service administration in relation to how Delafield Hospital could serve as an experience field for students. The participants were: the Director and Assistant Director of Nursing Education and Nursing Service of the Department of Hospitals; representatives of the Medical Board of Delafield Hospital (liaison between the Columbia-Presbyterian Medical Center and Delafield Hospital); the Director of the Division of Nursing Education of Teachers College and another Teachers College faculty member; the Director of the Nursing Service Administration projects of Teachers College.

After considerable explanation and discussion, the group agreed that cooperation of the three participating agencies was essential. The representatives of these three participating organizations—Delafield Hospital, a governmental agency; Columbia-Presbyterian Medical Center, a voluntary agency; and Teachers College, Columbia University, a private agency—all pledged their support to the nursing and nursing service administration projects. They agreed that Delafield Hospital would be used as a Teaching Demonstration Center, for the purposes of this study.

The Director of the Nursing Service of Delafield Hospital was appointed to the staff of Teachers College as a part-time field supervisor.

A Project Planning Group was set up, including primarily staff members of the Division of Nursing Education of Teachers College and the Director of Nursing Service of Delafield Hospital. This group maintained a cooperative relationship throughout the development of the study. In the beginning, the Director of Nurses was the only representative of the nursing service, since her staff was not appointed until after the opening of the hospital. Inclusion of the rest of the nursing service staff was partially accomplished in the employment interview, at which time the Director of Nurses interpreted the projected plans for the cooperative development of Delafield as a demonstration center.

Over-all plans for the organization of nursing teams in Delafield Hospital were formulated. Final details of planning and actual procedures were, however, delayed until such time as nursing service personnel were available to participate in the project. Advance planning with the nursing service staff insured the participation and cooperation of its members throughout the study.

The mutual concern of the educational institution and the service agency was the need for improvement in the nursing care program of hospitals in general. It was envisioned that the projected study would provide an opportunity to set up a research field in which it would be possible to break away from traditional practice and seek ways of improving nursing care.

As has been said, contractual agreements provided for the development of the nursing service of Delafield Hospital on a nursing team basis. It was agreed that orientation of nursing service personnel and assistance in organizing the nursing service were to be assumed by the project staff of the Division of Nursing Education. The facilities of the cooperating hospital were made available to the project staff and to students of the Division of Nursing Education for concurrent participation in action research toward the direct improvement of the bedside nursing care of its patients.

Although the cooperating hospital was new in terms of structure, it was in actuality part of an established institution: the organization of the departments would function according to the routines, policies, and procedures of the Department of Hospitals. This was an important factor in the experimentation, for it provided an opportunity to study the effect of change and the methodology involved in the reorganization of a nursing service on a team basis.

Any proposals for the improvement of nursing service should be adaptable to the large number of hospitals already in existence. Although this study concerns itself primarily with reorganization, the results are equally applicable to the organization of a new institution. However, the true value of the nursing team approach must be measured in terms of its adaptability to the average nursing service department. In the development of the nursing service of Delafield Hospital on a nursing team basis, within the organizational framework of the Department of Hospitals, the emphasis fell on reorganization.

It was recognized that a general hospital might find the implications of this study limited, inasmuch as it was conducted in a specialized service, the cooperating hospital being a 309-bed hospital for treatment and research in the care of patients with cancer and allied diseases.

Cancer is the second cause of death in the United States. It attacks all age groups and invades all organs and tissues of the body. Medical therapy for cancer includes surgical intervention, X-ray and radiation therapy, and chemotherapy. It is a basic assumption that there are common elements in nursing care of all patients, regardless of the health problem or the environment. This is carried further to the recognition of the fact that there are common elements in the care of patients whose health problems are associated with a particular organ. Thus, what is true of the nursing activities in a specialized service will in varying degree be true of the generalized service or hospital.

The scope of the clinical situation does not affect a study of the role of the professional nurse as a team leader, for the competencies of the team leader are those required of a professional nurse in *any* situation.

The nursing profession's knowledge of a particular health problem or group of health problems is continuously supplemented through individual study, participation in advanced educational programs, and participation in in-service educational programs.

The assignment of a nurse's aide or a practical nurse to the nursing team enhanced this study. The patient's and family's emotional reaction to cancer accentuated the need for some understanding of the patient's problems by *all* personnel having direct contact with the patient and his family. This need was integral to the planning of how best to prepare nonprofessional personnel for the team.

The date of February 1, 1951, was set for the opening of Delafield Hospital. One month before that date, two members of the College project staff went to the Delafield Hospital and participated actively in all of the detailed planning for the organization of the nursing teams, the orientation of nursing personnel, the compilation of administrative procedures, the physical placement of supplies and equipment on the ward units, the development of an on-the-job training program, in-service programs, and the like.

It was in this initial planning phase that students first participated in the activities of the Teaching Demonstration Center. All students majoring in nursing service administration in the Division of Nursing Education were invited by the nursing service staff to visit the hospital and to suggest plans for the organization of the nursing service units. Members of the Delafield nursing service and of the College project staff worked with groups of these students to develop plans for the following units: the out-patient department, the central supply room, the operating room, the head nurse station, a patient unit, the treatment room, the utility room, and storage space.

The cooperative relationship which was noticeable from the beginning, between the hospital nursing service staff and the students and instructional staff of Teachers College, was to continue throughout the development of the Teaching Demonstration Center.

After the hospital officially opened in February, 1951, and it was evident that one ward unit at a time would be activated, one member of the College project staff was assigned the over-all responsibility for assisting the nursing service staff with the organization, on a team basis. The project staff as a whole, and other members of the instructional staff of the Division of Nursing Education, continued to participate and contribute to the over-all development of the Teaching Demonstration Center.

The development of the Teaching Demonstration Center on a nursing team basis was the result of the cooperative efforts of the entire nursing service staff of the hospital, the instructional staff of the Division of Nursing Education, and the many students who participated through field experience. From February, 1951 to June, 1953, 301 students participated in the study by means of field experience in nursing service administration, supervision, teaching of medical-surgical nursing and through one of the major courses in the prespecialization program, Relationships and Team Functions in Nursing.

This written report encompasses not only the findings of two studies —the early study by Leino (36) and the one which took the form of the development of the Teaching Demonstration Center on a nursing team basis—but also the experiences of other hospitals and basic schools of nursing in their development of the nursing service on a team basis, as met by the writer in working with them.

Although this report is intended as a guide, it is fully appreciated that adaptation of principles to any particular hospital must be made by the nursing service department of that hospital.

2. THE PROFESSIONAL HEALTH TEAM

THE PROFESSIONAL health team functions in the home, hospital, or other health agencies. The composition of the team is governed by the patient's health problems and the degree to which the patient is dependent upon others for assistance in the solution of his problem. Members of the team are the patient and his family, the physician, the graduate nurse, the social worker, the nutritionist, the clergyman, the occupational therapist, the physical therapist, and other allied professional workers.

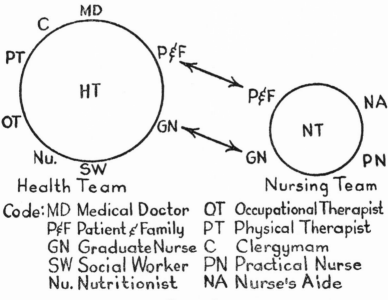

Health Team   Nursing Team

Code: MD Medical Doctor   OT Occupational Therapist
P&F Patient & Family   PT Physical Therapist
GN Graduate Nurse   C Clergymam
SW Social Worker   PN Practical Nurse
Nu. Nutritionist   NA Nurse's Aide

FIGURE 1

The physician is the leader of the professional health team. Responsibility for certain aspects of the total medical care plan is delegated by the physician to the other members. It is clearly recognized that each member has a unique function and that these functions relate to the whole plan of care for the individual patient.

The contributions of the various members of the health team may vary, with members assuming more or less active roles, depending upon the response of the patient or the complexity of his problems. The patient's response to illness is influenced by many factors. The major problem of the patient at the time medical therapy is indicated may not be his immediate physical health. It may be some basic emotional problem which interferes with his cooperation in the projected plan of medical therapy. An example will illustrate how the professional health team helps patients deal more effectively with their problems.

Mr._____, forty-two years old, was admitted to the hospital for biopsy and removal of a tumor of the jaw. He experienced the routine admission procedure of a busy ward and spent the remainder of the day in the solarium with other ambulatory patients. The report to the afternoon staff mentioned his routine preparation for surgery, and that he was ambulatory. This in turn was reported to the night staff.

During the night, Mr._____ slept very little; he walked to the bathroom frequently and was sitting in the chair at his bedside at 3 A.M.

The care of Mr._____'s bed was first assigned to a nurse's aide (he took his own bath and received no treatments or medications at this time), but a revision in assignment was made. A graduate nurse was charged with his care, upon the report of the night nurse and upon observation that Mr._____ was sitting at his bedside staring into space and not entering into the general activity of the ward. His breakfast tray was untouched except for the coffee. When the nurse's aide came into the ward to collect trays he asked her to remove his, stating that he was not hungry.

The assignment of the graduate nurse member of the nursing team had included the giving of baths to two patients in this ward. The making of Mr._____'s bed was included as a potential means for establishing direct contact with the patient.

The graduate nurse was interested in the opportunities in a ward for group teaching, and for establishing a functional relationship with patients other than those for whom she was providing direct physical care. It had been her experience that initial rapport was facilitated in certain instances if she was engaged in any small service to the patient. Once established, the relationship continued to develop, regardless of the involvement of the graduate nurse in providing direct physical care.

The graduate nurse, on entering the ward, visited with each patient and discussed his plans for the day; this included mention of the names of personnel who would participate in his care. In approaching Mr. _____, she told him that she would be the one to make his bed and when, approximately, she would be with him.

During the morning activity, Mr.＿＿ gradually entered into the general conversation of the ward, and when the graduate nurse returned to make his bed he spoke freely to her about his family. In reviewing his record the nurse had noted that he was married and had four children ages six to fourteen; he was a salesman; owned his own home; was in excellent physical condition except for the tumor; and had claimed no religious affiliation.

At one point Mr.＿＿ asked the nurse when she was to be off duty for the day. Upon hearing that it was Friday, he remarked that he probably wouldn't be around when she returned. This was Tuesday and he was scheduled for operation on Friday. The patient further revealed to the nurse that he anticipated death during or following surgery.

When he signed the operative permit, on admission to the hospital, he was apparently cooperating, but in fact the decision for surgery had been made for him, not with him.

The patient's conversation with the nurse and other nursing service personnel, their observation of his behavior, analysis of his record, and contact with his wife during visiting hours implied several factors which might have influenced his reaction. The nurse conferred with the physician, and at a conference which included the social worker the following questions were raised for further exploration: What were his feelings toward life? Toward death? What was his usual response to problems in his normal life situation? What were his feelings associated with the tumor growth? Did he anticipate a diagnosis of cancer? If so, did he believe that death was an inevitable sequela of cancer? Did he believe that pain was inescapable? How important was his physical appearance? Did he anticipate that a change in his physical appearance or a possible disfigurement would affect family relationships? Was he apprehensive about the effect of a possible disfigurement on his work as a salesman? Would the surgery affect his family income? What effect, if any, did religion have on his apparent acceptance of death following surgery? Did relationships within the family group affect his response? What previous experiences with doctors, hospitals, or illness might have influenced his response?

The physician, social worker, and nurse, guided by these questions, stressed the importance of accurate observation and reporting by any and all personnel having contact with Mr.＿＿. Plans for surgery were delayed.

The major objective of the health team at this time was to assist the patient to express his feelings concerning the projected surgery, to revise the plan of care in the light of these responses, and to foster his active participation in the new plan.

The relationship of the patient and nurse was such that the nurse continued to assume a major role in this aspect of therapy.

Following the second conference of the physician, social worker, and nurse, the priest was notified. (The nurse had noticed a rosary in the drawer of Mr._____'s bedside table.)

While visiting other patients in the ward, the priest stopped and greeted Mr._____ but did not discuss religion. Later, Mr._____ told the nurse that he was surprised that the priest hadn't talked about religion or even asked him his faith, and that he seemed to be a regular fellow. A natural discussion of religion resulted, with the other patients entering in. Mr._____ commented that he hoped the priest would stop by again.

The priest, notified of this by the nurse, visited the ward again the next day. Mr._____ followed him outside the ward and said that someday he would like to talk to him privately. The priest immediately led him to an unoccupied room and they talked for well over an hour. At the conclusion of the conference, Mr._____ told the nurse he wanted to see the doctor.

In the meantime, the priest had had a conference with the physician.

When the doctor arrived, the patient, for the first time, asked direct questions about the surgery involved. Indirectly he had questioned the nurse, but with the physician he had assumed a submissive role. The possibility of the tumor's being benign or malignant was discussed and the resulting surgery for either diagnosis was explained, with Mr._____ probing for detailed information. At one point he said he had never realized that doctors told patients anything, and that he was a man who liked to face facts. The end result was the scheduling of the operation by the physician and patient jointly.

This case illustrates the interdependence of the members of the health team in the total plan of medical care for a patient. Several problems were identified by the patient and, through the guidance of the professional personnel, the patient took the initiative in solving his own problems. Teamwork was the vehicle for achieving these results, and the patient was a recognized member of the team.

No attempt has been made to discuss the problems of this particular patient in detail. The method and the results are the important factors in this illustration.

3. THE NURSING TEAM

BY TEAM SPIRIT, we mean the desire to join forces with others in working toward a common goal.

By *teamwork,* we mean the smoothly coordinated and synchronized activity that characterizes a closely-knit group. It is based on: (1) team spirit in all members, (2) of a small group, (3) each of whom is able to make a practical contribution to the common goal, (4) who have frequent and full two-way communication in face-to-face talk to plan and evaluate group activity, and (5) continued practice in supplementing each other as team members.

If any of these elements is weak or lacking, teamwork is less effective than it might be. (53:84)

Relationship to Professional Health Team

Figure 1 (page 7) illustrates the relationship of the nursing team to the professional health team. The patient and his family and the graduate nurse are constants, and function as liaisons between the two teams. The interprofessional health team concerns itself with the total medical care plan of the patient; intraprofessional teams concern themselves with that aspect of the plan which is a delegated responsibility, or a recognized function of a particular professional group.

The Function of Nursing

Before any further discussion of the nursing team, it might be well to contemplate the function of nursing itself. Nursing is unique, its uniqueness lying in the close and individualized service to the patient, a service which may vary with his state of health from one of dependence in which the nurse performs for him what he cannot do for himself, through supportive and rehabilitative care, physical and emotional, to self-direction of his own health. (46:21)

Peplau develops a concept of nursing which complements the above definition.

Nursing is a significant, therapeutic, interpersonal process. It functions cooperatively with other human processes that make health possible for individuals in communities. In specific situations in which a professional health team offers health services, nurses participate in the organization of conditions that facilitate natural ongoing tendencies in human organisms. Nursing is an educative instrument, a maturing force, that aims to promote

11

forward movement of personality in the direction of creative, constructive, productive, personal and community living. (49:16)

Philosophy of Nursing Team Organization and Functioning

The functioning nursing team is more than a reorganization or restructuring of a nursing service. It represents a philosophy of nursing and of patient care as well as a method of organization.

The nursing service department is one of the administrative units of the hospital through which the purposes of the institution are carried out. The pattern of organization adopted by the nursing service department should be one which enables it to fulfill its purpose in a cooperative functioning relationship with other departments of the hospital. The primary function of the hospital is to care for the sick and injured. Other important functions, such as cooperation in the education of physicians, nurses, and other personnel, and in research, are subordinate and are recognized as part of the responsibility of the hospital because they contribute indirectly to the care of the sick.

The scope of nursing in the care of the sick and injured covers a range of activities directly influenced by the nurse-patient and nurse-family relationship. This is a significant factor in the provision of nursing care by the nursing team. Since the purpose of the nursing department is nursing service to patients, the needs of the patient determine the services to be provided. The patient is the hub of activity and, nursing service personnel functions are defined to accomplish the necessary services. Policies and routines are determined and influenced by the type of service provided as well as by the quality of service the nursing personnel wish to provide.

The development of policies concerned with patient services begins with a consideration of the patient and his needs. For example, visiting hours are a common "problem." What is the purpose of visiting hours? All too often they become barriers and appear to further the separation of the patient from his family. If the nursing service department and hospital administration are concerned with the patient as a member of a family and are aware of the need for planning with the family, policies concerning visiting hours will be influenced accordingly.

Hospital policies, rules and regulations reflect the philosophy of the various departments. Two distinct groups of people exist in the hospital: patients and personnel. Certain policies are directly concerned with personnel; others are directly concerned with patient and family services. Those concerned with the patient and family services should not be unduly affected by hospital routines or pressures of service. Again using the same example, are visiting-hour policies influenced by service needs of personnel or those of patients? Is there a relationship between the service needs of personnel and the needs of patients and families which affects the development of policies? Is it a question of whether the nurse perceives her role as doing for and deciding for, or doing with and deciding with, the patient?

In the study of nursing team organization and functioning, the organization of the nursing service started with the patient and those in direct contact with the patient—the nursing team. The character and quality of service were defined and the relationship of other personnel and services to the over-all purpose was identified. This philosophy is clearly demonstrated by reversing the general pattern of organizational charts. (See Figure 2.)

Rank, as such, is nonexistent within the team membership or within the total organization of the nursing service. It is unfortunate if team relationship gives the connotation of gradations of rank, for a profession dependent upon position for its security is subject to limitation in the continuous process of development. Authority is inherent, but it is an authority which recognizes the individual's potential and maintains an environment in which he contributes to the height of his potential. The real authority of the situation is the patient and his nursing needs.

Responsibility for a part of the total medical care plan is delegated to the professional nurse. As team leader, she recognizes that authority is necessarily associated with professional responsibility, and that the contributions of all nursing service personnel are affected by the preparation of the individual for his role. Guidance in the provision of nursing service through professional leadership provides for a cohesion of otherwise isolated activities and personnel. Within team relationships, authority loses the connotation of power and takes on a meaning of control—control which is recognized and developed within the group.

Members of the Nursing Team

On the ward unit of the average hospital three groups of nursing service personnel, with wide variation of preparation and experience, are potential members of the nursing team. Following is a list of nursing service personnel, with explanatory material.

Graduate nurses or general staff nurses

The basic nursing curriculum may be three, four or five years in length. The three-year program is for the most part conducted by a

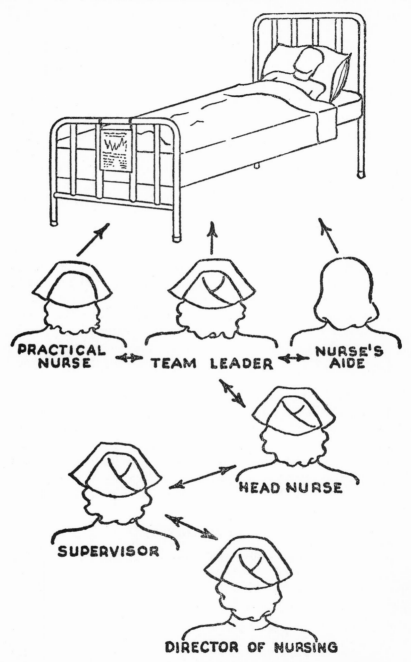

FIGURE 2. A PHILOSOPHY OF NURSING SERVICE ORGANIZATION

hospital school of nursing. The four- or five-year programs which lead to a degree are established in colleges, universities, or hospitals in connection with degree-granting institutions. Examination of the learning experiences provided in the various programs reveals the diversity of preparation. Some may have supplemented their basic education by attendance at an educational institution or through work experience.

Private duty nurses

These are graduate nurses who have been employed by the patient, as differentiated from the general staff nurse employed by the hospital.

Practical nurses

The educational program for practical nurses is established in vocational schools or in hospitals and is, for the most part, of a year's duration. In states where licensure is mandatory, applicants may be licensed by waiver, upon certification of experience. A large proportion have had no preparation other than experience in the work situation. Employment practices are not uniform, and therefore experience in one hospital situation does not insure preparation for practice in another. Programs in the various schools differ so widely that there is great diversity in preparation. In certain instances a practicing nurse may be a former student who had withdrawn from a basic program for graduate nurses.

Auxiliary personnel

This group includes nurse's aides, orderlies, hospital attendants, and others who may or may not have had previous hospital experience. Some hospitals provide an organized, on-the-job training program; others depend on orientation from the personnel of the ward unit to which the newcomer has been assigned.

Red Cross nurse's aides

This is a volunteer group which provides patient care in some hospitals. All have a uniform preparation and supervised practice period before being assigned to a hospital to become part of the nursing service.

The increasing ratio of nonprofessional to professional nursing service personnel in the average patient unit has tended to dilute the services provided. A review of the types of personnel involved, and of their wide range of preparation, is necessary for an understanding of the problems inherent in providing individualized patient care. The team method is a safeguard in the assignment and supervision of personnel. The hospital's responsibility in preparing the various types of personnel for membership on the nursing team is discussed later.

Differentiation of Function

Nursing team organization and functioning are based upon the philosophy that the individual patient and his problems are the point of departure and upon the assumption that there exists, within the scope of nursing, a differentiation of function.

The functions of nursing may be conceived of as being of a spectrum range. Many functions involve the performance of skills and techniques varying in difficulty and complexity and extending on a continuum, from the simplest performed by the mother and others and easily picked up without training, to the most complex function demanding a very high degree of skill and expertness that can be developed only with considerable training. Many functions also demand judgment ranging from that based upon common knowledge to judgment that can be arrived at only by bringing to bear upon the professional problems pertinent knowledge from an extensive reservoir of scientific information derived from many fields of study. The functions at one extreme of the range of the spectrum, those demanding a high degree of skill and judgment, must be the responsibility of nurses whose educational preparation has been of a professional type. Nurses who perform these functions can be assumed to need and to possess the breadth of scientific information with which to do reflective thinking and to have developed their higher intellectual powers and habits of reasoning, judging, and drawing inferences about nursing problems. (12:54)

Montag has diagramed the concept of nursing functions on a continuum or as having a spectrum range. (43:6)

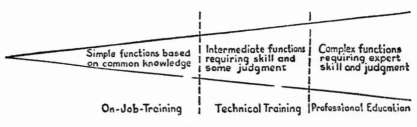

FIGURE 3

This concept illustrates the relationship of the three groups of workers. It is basic to nursing team organization and functioning. At the present time, nursing service personnel cannot be classified arbitrarily within the three divisions of the spectrum. The variation in preparation does result in overlapping but, in the process of the preparation for and in the actual functioning of the nursing team, shifts may often result. In-service education programs of the agency are a vital part of the process.

One end of the spectrum may be said to represent assisting functions—those which involve skills readily learned on the job, and also hygienic and homemaking functions such as those commonly taught to lay people in the Red Cross home nursing course.

In the middle section are the semiprofessional or technical functions. Included are duties required in the physical care of patients and in carrying out medical orders of the physician. The exercise of judgment must usually be restricted to those situations likely to be largely repetitive and routine, and handled under the supervision of a professional nurse or physician.

The other end of the spectrum would, then, represent the responsibility of the professional nurse. The symbolism of the diagram is the open-ended or limitless opportunities for the development of the profession of nursing, as compared to the rigid confines of a vocation. Requisite is an ability for the application of scientific principles to problem solving in planning, providing, and evaluating nursing care.

Using the concept illustrated in Figure 3, personnel can be evaluated for their role on the nursing team. Nurse's aides, orderlies, and other auxiliary workers are assigned simple functions, dependent upon their preparation. Practical nurses may be ready for no more than simple functions if their experience has been only on the job, or for some intermediate functions if they are graduates of a practical nurse program. The graduate nurse may be prepared to function in the intermediate area only, or she may function partially or entirely in the area requiring expert skill and judgment. The team leader must be capable of functioning in the complex area.

Method for Assignment of Patient Care

It is a misconception to believe that nursing team organization is merely a reorganization of the functional method, with the general staff nurse rather than the head nurse as team leader.

The case method and the functional method are recognized patterns of providing nursing service. In the case method, the total care of the patient is assigned to one member of the nursing service staff. With the functional method came a beginning recognition of a division of labor, with the emphasis on jobs to be done for the patient. These jobs are grouped in the interests of economy of time and expediency of service.

In the functional method of assignment it is common to find one person administering all medications, one taking all temperatures, and so forth.

Team nursing is, in actuality, a synthesis of case and functional method. It recognizes the changing role of the professional nurse in relation to the increasing number of nonprofessional personnel. It is an attempt to meet the increased demands for nursing service and is based on the philosophy that the individual patient is the deciding factor, and that all personnel having contact with the patient and his family share in and can contribute to the planning, providing, and evaluating of nursing care.

The case method as an over-all pattern of assignment is impossible when services of nonprofessional personnel are utilized for patient care. Total care of patients cannot and should not be assigned to other than the professional nurse, because nursing care is concerned with more than the technical aspects. Classification of patients into groupings such as subacute, convalescent, and chronic in order to facilitate assignment to practical nurses or nurse's aides is, for the most part, based on the physical response of the patient to his illness. Such classifications ignore the emotional and rehabilitative problems of the patient as well as the aspect of family health supervision. Assignment of individuals or groups of patients for total care to nonprofessional personnel can only result in routine care.

In the use of the functional method, the professional nurse tends to lose the intimate contact with patients. She becomes primarily concerned with treatments and medications or with only the acutely ill. This method can result in an assembly line approach, with the identity of the patient lost in the lists of jobs to be done. Certain groups of patients may have little or no contact with a professional nurse, the jobs to be done falling within the realm of the nonprofessional worker. The individual patient and his problems are overshadowed by orders and routines.

In the patient unit which employs the team method of nursing service, the head nurse is responsible for the over-all administration and supervision of the unit. She delegates to the team leader part of the responsibility for coordination and supervision of patient services.

The team leader is a general staff nurse, appointed by the head nurse, who has demonstrated competency in nursing practice and leadership ability, or perhaps a recognizable potential ability.

Cooperatively the head nurse and team leaders plan for assignment of personnel to the nursing team, and evaluate patients' nursing needs for grouping and assignment to specific teams.

The members of the team share in the responsibility for assignments within the team, but it is the leader who is ultimately responsible, with the supervision and assistance of the head nurse. Patients' nursing needs are evaluated in relation to the personnel available as team members. The groups of patients assigned to the nursing team and the team membership are parallel forces. In planning the assignment, the procedure is one of first identifying those patients or those phases of the nursing care plans which require professional judgment and skill. Following the professional nurse's or team leader's assignment, if she is the only professional nurse member of the team, a similar procedure is carried out for the practical nurses and auxiliary personnel. The wide variation in the preparation and ability of the nonprofessional personnel requires individual consideration of every assignment. Coordination of activities is assured by a clearly defined written plan which indicates the relationship of individual participating team members.

Insofar as possible, direct contacts with the patient are minimized in planning the assignments. The team leader establishes a direct relationship with all patients assigned to the team, although she may not be providing direct physical service. This necessitates two contacts in the situation where the nonprofessional member of the team is participating. It is the responsibility of the team leader to plan, in the case of each patient, for this personal contact with a professional nurse. As the patient develops from a state of dependence, physical or emotional, to direction of his own care, the need for, or the degree of, immediate supervision by a professional nurse is diminished.

Examination of a typical assignment to a nursing team reveals aspects of both functional and case methods. The nurse's aide may be assigned a number of beds to be made or assistance with bed baths. The graduate nurse may be assigned total responsibility for the nursing care of selected patients, or she may be assigned a functional area. For example, she may be responsible for the administration of medication, if it is hospital policy that medicines be administered by a graduate nurse and if she is the only graduate nurse on the team; or she may assume this activity merely as a means of contact with patients. Differences in assignment result from the relationships of the team members and from the supervision of the team leader.

Communication Within the Nursing Team

The team leader must be available to the team members, and provision must be made for frequent face-to-face contact of the various members of the team in order to plan and evaluate the nursing care.

Each day the nursing team has a conference to identify the problems of patients, as experienced by the members of the nursing team, and to evaluate and plan for the patients' nursing care.

As a result of the conference, and of the personal contact of members of the nursing team with patients, a written plan of care is developed for each patient. It is a continuous plan, begun upon admission of the patient, evaluated daily, and changed as the need arises. The written plan is a means of communication within the team and serves as the basis for assignment.

During and immediately following the nursing team conference, the nursing care plans are brought up to date. Assignments are then made out for the following day.

All members of the nursing service of one patient unit must attend and participate in exchange reports of the various shifts. Following this report, the leader meets with the other team members, and adjustments are made in the assignment if necessary. This permits any necessary clarification of assignment or exchange of contributions by the various members of the team to the immediate plan for the day.

Continuity for the Twenty-four Hour Period

All principles discussed in this chapter apply to the provision of nursing care for the twenty-four hour period. The scope of activity during the morning necessitates a larger staff than at any other part of the twenty-four hours, but the afternoon or night assignments do not negate team relationships. Assignment is based on differentiation of function, with the graduate nurse assuming the direct supervisory relationship as team leader. In certain circumstances her unit may be larger; for example, if one graduate covers two units at night. Continuity of care is provided by use and continued development of individual nursing care plans.

4. THE NURSING TEAM LEADER

THE TEAM LEADER, as has been said, is always a graduate nurse, appointed by the head nurse, who has demonstrated competence in nursing practice and leadership ability, or at least potential ability.

Role of the Team Leader

The major responsibility of the team leader can be stated in a few sentences. It is to plan, with the members of the team, the nursing care required by a group of patients assigned to the team; to direct and supervise the members of the nursing team in carrying out the plan; to participate in the provision of nursing care; and to provide a means whereby the team continuously evaluates and revises the plan to meet the changing needs of the patient.

Basically, the team leader is a practitioner, participating in direct patient care. It is not intended that the emphasis of her role should be administrative.

The knowledge, skills, abilities, attitudes, and values essential to the practitioner are equally essential for effective leadership of a team, in any nursing situation. The practitioner who "works alone" and limits her activities to "my patients" or "my assignment" fails to recognize the sphere of influence of nursing. A nurse, whether on a team or not, never works alone. On the contrary, she has a cooperative relationship with other health professions. Also, in order to execute a distinctive function of nursing—that of assisting the individual and family to develop from dependence to self-direction—she must work with the family as well as the patient.

The title of team leader gives no guarantee that the leadership will be accepted by the group, for the success of team functioning depends to a large extent upon the quality of leadership. The loyalty and effectiveness of the group must be earned. This fact has proved difficult for many graduate nurses to accept. The hierarchy within the hospital has promoted the passing of orders or directions down the line; rarely has any influence seeped upward from the practical nurse or the nurse's aide. Thus, it will be seen that the act of organizing a nursing service on a team basis, even though a fairly simple procedure, does not necessarily insure team functioning of that team. The smoothly coordinated activity that characterizes a closely knit group is developed only through the acceptance of a group goal, and through the personal desire of its members to work together to accomplish that goal.

A primary factor in successful leadership is the leader's belief in the philosophy of the nursing team, and in the confidence she feels in her ability as a leader. She is in a position to foster increased personal satisfaction for team members. Cooperation is enlisted and participation gained only when the satisfactions derived from working as a unit outweigh the satisfactions of working alone. The organized nursing team is a safeguard of nursing services because it is the team itself which establishes goals of patient care and acts as a check and balance by means of continuous evaluation. Use of the team method is a conscious effort to utilize the forces which induce job satisfactions, thereby improving nursing care by providing opportunities for continuous growth of personnel.

Basic to the development of nursing teams and the role of the team leader is the acceptance of the "Assumptions of the Functions of Nursing" outlined by R. Louise McManus. (12:54) The functions of the professional nurse are presented as fundamental to the practice of nursing and therefore to the team leader. These assumptions are proposed as a basis for discussion.

The function of the professional nurse is conceived to parallel somewhat that of the professional physician. The unique responsibility of the physician recognized by law is to identify the medical problem, diagnose, and plan and prescribe treatment Although the physician carries out some of the treatment and the ultimate responsibility for it all remains his, he may delegate responsibility for some of the treatment to members of related professions, such as nurses, dietitians, physical therapists, or he may delegate responsibility even to the patient and his family, provided he is confident that they are capable of carrying out the treatment effectively and with safety. Similarly, the unique function of the professional nurse may be conceived to be:

1. The identification or diagnosis of the *nursing* problem and the recognition of its many interrelated aspects.

2. The deciding upon a course of nursing action to be followed for the solution of the problem, in the light of immediate and long-term objectives of nursing, with regard to prevention of illness, direct care, rehabilitation, and promotion of the highest standard of health possible for the individual.

3. The development with the assistance of other members of the nursing and health team, both intraprofessional and interprofessional, of a satisfactory plan of nursing care, including therapeutic, preventive, and rehabilitative measures, and treatments for which the physician has delegated responsibility to the nurse.

4. The continued direction of the program of nursing toward its optimum accomplishment, with adjustments in the plan as the nature of the problem changes, and the performance of those aspects which demand expert skill and judgment.

5. The progressive evaluation of the process and the results of nursing for the continuous improvement of the care of the patient and the practice of nursing.

These assumptions imply an ability on the part of the professional nurse to be self-directive; knowledge of and ability to apply scientific principles influencing nursing care; ability to employ problem-solving techniques; skill and ability in the techniques of interpersonal relationships including communication—all of which are fundamental to the ability to plan, provide, and evaluate individualized nursing care.

In her role of team leader, the competence or ability of the professional nurse practitioner is accentuated. As a member of the nursing team, her relationships are direct and as team leader she directly influences the quality of nursing care and of group relationships. The group develops only insofar as the quality of leadership fosters growth.

For the team leader, Leino has outlined the following essential steps in planning, directing, giving, and evaluating patient-centered care. (35)

Identify the patient's nursing problems.

Interpret nursing problems to co-workers and seek their cooperation in planning.

Formulate and record the nursing care plan.

Differentiate and delegate all aspects of nursing care.

Direct the program of nursing care.

Evaluate and record the results of nursing care.

Each step requires analysis to identify the abilities, skills, knowledge, and values the professional nurse requires to function as a team leader.

Identifying the Patient's Nursing Problem

In all too many situations nursing has consisted of carrying out doctors' orders and fulfilling certain hospital routines, such as baths. Nursing problems differ for each patient. Both the clinical diagnosis and the plan of medical therapy influence the plan of nursing care, but the major problems of the patient depend upon the patient as a person and upon his total experiences, his relationship and role in the family, and his response both physically and emotionally to the disease process and to the plan of medical therapy.

For example, Mary S＿＿＿ was admitted to the hospital for removal of a breast tumor. She was fifteen years old, and the oldest of five children. Mary's parents were born in Italy and the family's present home was in an Italian settlement in New York. Upon admission Mary requested a note for her school teacher explaining her hospitalization and consequent absence, but stated she did not want the diagnosis mentioned. Mary's mother was present but her only response was a shrug of the shoulders. The immediate nursing problem was to help Mary explore her emotional reaction to the lump in her breast. Analysis of the problem by the nurse identified the following factors, and raised the accompanying questions, regarding Mary's attitude.

Mary was in the adolescent group. (What were the facts about adolescent growth and development which would help the nurse understand Mary?)

Mary was a member of a family and community group retaining the Italian culture. (Were her school experiences and home experiences compatible? What was Mary's role in the family as the oldest child? As a daughter? What was the mother's and father's attitude toward explaining growth and development of the female body to Mary?)

Mary was a sophomore in high school. (Did she attend school functions? Did she bring friends to her home? Did she participate in functions involving both sexes? Had she attended lectures on growth and development of the male and female?)

Mary was a Catholic. (What influence did religion have on Mary's response?)

Contact with the mother, father, and Mary herself clarified family relationships and attitudes. The cooperation of the mother was gained and her permission was obtained to discuss with Mary the physiological changes which were occurring in her body.

The developing relationship between the nurse and Mary permitted Mary to explore her feelings concerning the tumor. She was conscious that her breast development was more extensive than that of her friends. Her family did not permit her to "date" but she had gone to a movie with a boy, after telling her parents she was visiting a girl friend. Further exploration showed that guilt feelings were associated with the tumor, a growth which Mary thought of as a punishment for disobeying her parents.

Details of this nurse-patient relationship will not be discussed further here. Referral was made to the school nurse, following Mary's discharge.

This case is presented to demonstrate the problem-solving method used by a professional nurse in the identification of the patient's nursing problem. The cue was given by the patient. It happened to be a verbal cue but it could just as well have been nonverbal or behavioral in nature. The nurse, seeing the cue as the major problem, assisted the family and patient to recognize the problem and to work toward its solution.

Only with the resource of a body of knowledge which is based upon scientific principles can the nurse plan for, and provide, individualized nursing care. In providing nursing service for individuals and families in communities she needs a background in the sociological, physical, biological, and psychological sciences.

Skill in the techniques of problem-solving is another competence which is essential for the team leader.

Interpretation and Cooperation

Interpretation requires skill in the techniques of communication; the seeking of cooperation requires skill in the techniques of interpersonal relationships. Communication is recognized as an aspect of interpersonal relationships but is, for emphasis, identified separately. In both, judgment is a major component, for the problem is not only how to communicate but what to communicate and to whom.

The privacy of the patient is respected but some information must be shared between the professional nurse and the allied professional group. Judgment must be exercised as to the extent and nature of information which should be shared by the nonprofessional members.

Interpretation of the nursing problem is a sharing process, for in it are involved the reactions of the individuals concerned, and of the group as a whole, to their relationships with patients and families. Through personal contact each individual gains her own impressions of the needs of patients. The team leader must be capable of assimilating the varied communications of the members of the team; of identifying with the group those cues which have implications for nursing care; and of channeling the cues into positive action. The cues may reinforce or alter the plan of nursing care for the patient.

The team leader has the responsibility of drawing from her own experience, and of introducing pertinent information which she has secured from the patient, the family, the patient's record, or from other nursing or allied professional workers. Introduction of information into the group is in terms of its needs for the planning, providing, and evaluating of nursing care.

The team leader must be available for on-the-spot conferences with members of the nursing team. In many instances the capacity for anticipating needs is required until such time as personnel develop and demonstrate individually the capacity for self-evaluation.

A daily team conference is scheduled so that the entire team, through a discussion of the problems encountered, may evaluate past experience and plan future nursing care. In the majority of situations the afternoon has been the favorable time, since all personnel have had contact with patients and have carried out the major portion of the plan for the day. This time allows for meeting the patient's needs and for planning the following day's assignments as well as preparing the report to the next group.

The conference does not replace the face-to-face contact of a member of the nursing team and the team leader as the need arises. Details of the conference will be discussed in a separate chapter.

The morning, afternoon, or night report to the group on duty is another means of interpreting patients' nursing problems. Following the presentation of the report, which all members of the team attend, the leader discusses with the team implications for nursing care and alters assignments, taking into consideration the patient's condition and the absence of personnel.

Planning is a continuous process and includes both long term and immediate objectives. The plan evolves as the team leader identifies the nursing responsibility associated with the total medical care plan. and as the members of the nursing team contribute to the interpretation of patients' nursing needs.

Formulating and Recording the Nursing Care Plan

This is a means of insuring continuity of nursing care and communication within and between nursing teams. All members of the nursing team contribute to the plan but the actual recording is done by the professional nurse, inasmuch as it involves decision-making and the exercise of professional judgment. A description of the form for recording and details of formulating nursing care plans are given in Chapter 7.

This phase of the functions of the team leader emphasizes the need for ability and skill in the techniques of communication and the importance of a sound background in scientific principles.

Differentiating and Delegating Aspects of Nursing Care

Evaluation of nursing personnel and of patient's nursing needs are concomitant factors. The team leader must be aware of the potential and the background experience of the team members as well as informed about the hospital policies regulating the activities of each group. The individual patient and the preparation and ability of the individual members of the team are the deciding elements.

In differentiating between and delegating the various aspects of nursing care, it is important for the team leader to assure the personal contact of herself and other professional nurses with the patient. There is always the danger that in the assessment of patients' nursing needs the emphasis, for the professional nurse, will be primarily on the administration of certain procedures or on the direct care of only those patients who are classified as acutely ill.

The professional nurse is responsible for the nursing care of patients, and the act of delegating certain aspects does not negate this responsibility. She must have close personal contact with patients if she is to identify their nursing needs and evaluate their nursing care.

The rapid turnover of patients in certain types of services—early ambulation particularly—presents major problems to the professional nurse. The shorter contact with the patient is a challenge to the ability of the nurse which must be recognized.

Direct contact with all new admissions is essential if the professional nurse is to identify the patient's nursing problems and to develop an initial plan of nursing care. The first impression often colors the reaction of the patient to his entire hospital experience, and all too often the professional responsibility for the orientation of the patient is neglected.

The nursing care plans for individual patients are used as a guide in the delegation or assignment of aspects of nursing care to the members of the nursing team. The plans are concerned with both the physical and the emotional response of the patient.

The patient's total nursing needs are assessed by the team leader, and aspects of care are assigned to the professional nurse, the practical nurse, or the nurse's aide, depending upon the degree of adjustment of the individual patient and the relationship of the specific activity to the total plan. It is not the individual activity which is important but the patient's general condition and the purpose for which the activity is performed. For example, a colostomy irrigation following surgery is the professional nurse's responsibility. The emotional and physical adjustment of the patient to interference with normal body function, and the rehabilitation and associated teaching require professional knowledge, judgment, and skill. When the patient has acquired the degree of independence which permits him to assume responsibility for this aspect of his care, the practical nurse may be assigned to provide him with the necessary equipment and assistance. Similarly, the patient who is admitted to the hospital with a colostomy may be assigned to the professional nurse for an evaluation of his understanding, adjustment, and ability as it relates to nutrition, care of skin, elimination, and so on. The subsequent assignment is dependent upon the nurse-patient evaluation of his needs.

In some situations the team leader has found, following her day off, that the taking of morning temperature, pulse, and respiration of all patients in the group has been a means of assessing changes in their general condition, of meeting new patients, and of establishing a productive relationship with them. Visiting the patient in the regular morning round did not appear to produce the same results. The patients responded to her interest in visiting them, but the act of doing facilitated communication. This may have been related to the nurse's skill in the techniques of interviewing and to the fact that the nurse is generally more at ease when she is engaged in physical activity.

Spot checking or superficial observation of the activities of a member of the nursing team is an ineffective means of evaluating the assignment. The purpose or rationale behind the assignment must be identified. In one instance, a supervisor criticized a team leader for making an empty bed. The patient concerned had been admitted for diagnosis, and spent much of his time sitting in the chair at his bedside. He did not engage in ward activity, responding only to direct questioning. The team leader was attempting to foster a relationship with this patient, while seemingly her only concern was to make the bed. It was an indirect approach and proved to be effective. After a three-day period, the patient responded to her directly and the activity was delegated to a nurse's aide.

For certain patients the assignment of activities may be divided between team members. For example, a patient with a fracture of the femur may be assigned to the practical nurse for assistance with the bed bath, to the professional nurse for the teaching and supervising of exercises and crutch-walking. Another example might be the patient who is allowed out of bed for a period of time in the morning and afternoon. The bed bath of this patient may be assigned to the practical nurse, and the nurse's aide may be assigned the responsibility for making the empty bed at the time the patient is sitting in the chair.

The assignment is made out in detail for all members of the team by the team leader, with supervision by the head nurse. Several methods have been used. A master sheet with the names of the team members entered in separate columns appears to be the most economical of time. This allows the team leader and the head nurse to check the assignment with the Kardex, and to get an overview of the activities of all members. The assignment is made out in the afternoon, revised after the morning report, and then entered by the individual team members in 3″ x 5″ notebooks which they carry in the pockets of their uniforms. In the early stages of development of this plan, assignments were entered in the individual notebooks by the team leaders, but this proved too time-consuming.

Such a detailed written assignment is a valuable safeguard in communication. The individual members of the team record in their notebooks any observations, results of nursing care, questions of patients, or other pertinent data. These notebooks are then used as a basis of discussion at the nursing team conference, and for reference in keeping the patient's chart. (See Exhibit I, page 82, for a sample assignment sheet.)

The head nurse makes assignments of groups of patients to a specific team for a minimum of one week for continuity of care, keeping a balance between admissions and discharges and the work load of a team, in terms of patients' nursing needs. It is preferable, for continuity of care, that patients and the team remain stable for the length of hospitalization of the patient. But it must be recognized that under certain circumstances, such as absence of a team member, special ability of team members, or a change in patient's condition, it may be desirable or necessary to make a change.

Directing and Participating in Nursing Care

The team leader is a member of the nursing team and as such participates in the provision of nursing care. She assumes the administrative responsibility of assignment to and supervision of the team, in addition to her function as a practitioner. This is a delegation of responsibility by the head nurse; it is not a matter of the head nurse's relinquishing responsibility, but of her sharing with and supervising the team leader in this activity. Direct supervision by the team leader is a practical approach to the problems resulting from the participation of the nonprofessional group in nursing service. Their immediate supervision is provided by a person who is active in the care of the patient, the general staff nurse.

Ability and skill in the techniques of interpersonal relationships are essential for the team leader. Basic should be the belief of the team leader in the worth of the contribution of the individual members of the team. Leadership is more than the issuing of orders; it calls for the ability to develop within the group situations which foster personal growth resulting in a willingness to assume responsibility. Discipline which is self-initiated is a safeguard. As each member contributes to the total plan, within an organizational pattern which permits her to contribute to the height of her potential, she experiences satisfaction and recognizes the limitations of her contribution. Thus the control of the plan comes from the group, with guidance from the team leader.

Evaluating the strengths and weaknesses of the individual members of the team and assisting them to develop a capacity for self-evaluation are continuous processes for the team leader.

Frequent demands are made upon the team leader for on-the-spot teaching of personnel. This is in addition to the teaching involved as a practitioner in patient care and is another phase of her responsibility in providing guidance or direction.

The team leader must be available to the members of the team. This does not imply a hovering relationship, but a readiness and willingness to participate in the solution of problems. It means attitudinal as well as physical proximity. The team leader is attitudinally available if the team members are familiar with her assignment as well as their own and if she is capable of evaluating the immediate needs of the total situation. Availability is often a selective procedure. A problem of the team member and the current activity of the team leader at that time are assessed to determine the relative urgency of the problems. A joint decision stimulates the feeling of availability, although assistance may be postponed temporarily.

Evaluating and Recording Results of Nursing Care

Evaluation is a continuous process. Identification of nursing problems and formulation of both nursing objectives and definite plans of nursing care provide tangible means of evaluation. The daily nursing team conference provides a means for all members to participate in the evaluation of patient responses to the plan.

The patient is always the indicator of the success of a plan for his nursing care. It is his response and personal involvement which determine the effectiveness of the results.

Recording is an essential element of evaluation, for it provides a progress report of both the development and the fulfillment of the plan. It is a means of communication between members of the nursing service and allied professional groups, the nursing plan being only one phase of the total medical care plan. The recording of the progress of the patient, as experienced by the nursing team, provides an instrument for evaluation of the plan of nursing care as it relates to the total plan of medical care.

Nurses' notes, if they assume the character of evaluations, are progress notes. Recording is objective, concise, and anecdotal in nature.

Summary

Administration of nursing care for a group of patients involves the functions of planning, organizing, directing, coordinating, controlling, and evaluating. The team leader supervises the members of the nursing team in the provision of nursing care and is responsible for teaching patients and families, as well as for teaching members of the nursing team. These functions are in addition to the direct care of patients by the team leader and are presented as a summary of the scope of functions of the team leader.

5. THE HEAD NURSE

NURSING TEAMS and team leadership do not negate the supervisory relationship of the head nurse to the nursing service personnel. The complexity of problems in the average patient unit, influenced by the increasing proportion of nonprofessional to professional workers, has increased the demands for supervision.

The head nurse is the coordinator of patient services of the hospital unit. Her chief function as administrator of the ward unit is the maintenance of a total environment conducive to the best possible nursing care. She is primarily concerned with people: patients, visitors, family, personnel. Her administrative functions include the provision or facilitation of services so that the combined efforts of personnel may result in proper nursing care of patients. The leadership role of the head nurse requires immediate and sustained contact with the entire nursing service staff of the unit. It is through the process of supervision that this contact with personnel is productive, for both personnel and patients. Supervision, then, is a relationship between two or more people; a cooperative relationship which stimulates growth of the person being supervised, thereby increasing efficiency.

Relationship to Team Leader

The head nurse identifies potential team leaders in the general staff nurse group and assists them in the development of abilities and skills necessary to the functions of the team leader. The general staff nurses are and have been functioning as practitioners. Additional skill and ability are required in the field of administration, supervision, and teaching. The head nurse delegates responsibility to the general staff nurse when the latter demonstrates a potential for assuming this responsibility as team leader.

The concentrated supervisory effort of the head nurse with the team leaders or graduate nurse staff insures a continuity of supervision for the nonprofessional members of the nursing team in the immediate patient environment. The head nurse still maintains direct contact with patients and personnel in the unit. The team leader functions as a liaison—not as a block in organization hierarchy.

Coordination of Patient Services

The medical care plan of the patient is a guide to the plan for professional services. This plan and the professional services provided by the hospital determine the numbers and involvement of professional personnel other than medical and nursing.

A variety of services is centered in the patient unit. Ancillary services such as housekeeping and maintenance are examples of non-professional but necessary services which affect the control of the patient's environment. These services require the active participation, within the ward unit, of other groups of workers.

The head nurse, in cooperation with other department heads and allied professional groups, develops a plan for the coordination and provision of patient services. Without planning, and provision for follow-up, the emphasis of each group of workers is on the job to be done rather than on the relationship of the job to patient services.

Participation as a Member of the Health Team

The head nurse is the continuous representative of the nursing service personnel on the professional health team. It is she who is ultimately responsible for identifying the nursing responsibilities in the total plan of medical care. Plans may concern one patient or a group of patients and may have immediate or long-term implications for nursing. Continuity in planning for nursing service is insured by the participation of the head nurse.

Team leaders and general staff nurses also participate as members of the professional health team in planning, evaluating, and providing nursing care for patients assigned to their nursing team.

Evaluation of Patients' Nursing Needs

The head nurse is responsible for providing nursing care for patients on the unit and for supervising that care. The grouping of patients for assignment to nursing teams and the supervision of the plan of nursing care require continuous evaluation. This presupposes that the head nurse will have direct contact with patients. Through her immediate and sustained contact with patients she is able to assist the team leader to identify patients' nursing needs and to develop a plan of assignment which will help the patient to meet these needs.

Evaluation and Assignment of Personnel

In assigning personnel to teams, the head nurse assists the team leader to evaluate the potential and actual contribution of each member. Supervisory needs are identified as a result of the relationship of the head nurse and the team leader to the members of the nursing team, and plans are developed to meet these needs. This process includes measurement of the scope of responsibility of the individual team leader and self-evaluation on her part.

Assignment of nursing service personnel includes provision of coverage for the ward unit. Time off is provided for within the team.

Provision for Continuity of Nursing Care

The nursing team functions for the total twenty-four hour period. The head nurse is responsible for insuring continuity of nursing service within the unit and within the service of the hospital. In this responsibility she is assisted by the leader and other members of the team. If the patient goes to the operating room or for X ray, continuity in his total plan of nursing care must be provided.

Revision of Grouping of Patients

As the condition of patients changes, or as they are admitted or discharged, a revision of assignment is decided upon jointly by the head nurse and the team leader.

Revision of Composition of Nursing Teams

As nursing service personnel are employed, resign, take vacations or leaves of absence, go on sick leave, are rotated to day, afternoon, or night duty, or are transferred within the hospital, revisions are made in the assignment of personnel to nursing teams. At times a change in nursing team membership may be desirable because of some personality difference on the part of patient or staff.

Evaluation of Quality of Nursing Service

As has been said, the functioning nursing team carries on continuous evaluation of the effectiveness of service provided by its members. The head nurse actively engages in all aspects of evaluation, assisting the team leaders and other team members in an over-all appraisal of the effectiveness of the care as planned and provided.

Identification of Nursing Service Problems Needing Study

The head nurse is continuously concerned with the improvement of nursing service. She identifies nursing service problems which need study and plans cooperatively with nursing and other hospital personnel for the solution of these problems.

6. THE NURSING TEAM CONFERENCE

THE CONFERENCE is the nucleus of the in-service nursing program. At the conference there spring up spontaneously many teaching opportunities which are invaluable in terms of the application to specific patient problems. Techniques of group process and principles of interpersonal relationship are an integral part of the procedure. Observations made during a nursing team conference offer unique opportunities for guidance of nursing service personnel.

Conference Procedure

A time is planned each day for the members of the nursing team to meet as a group. During this period patients' problems are identified and explored, and an approach is developed by the team. The nursing care plans are revised or further developed, according to the changing needs of patients.

Each member of the nursing team has recorded during the course of the day the response of the patient to her care, the worker's observations of the patient, and questions or comments of the patient. These individual notes are used as guides in conference.

The team leader, using the Kardex as a guide, reads the patient's name and the objective of nursing care. The members of the nursing team who have contact with the patient discuss his response to his care and any additional information which may have been gained through contact with him or his family. Problems are identified by the group, and a plan is projected for the solution of the problems. The Kardex is revised by the team leader at this time. The objective is altered if new problems indicate a change in approach. Problems which are no longer evident are crossed out.

The head nurse functions as a resource person and assists the team leader and the team members in identifying nursing problems and developing nursing care plans.

The nursing team conference is the planning stage for the team, and the assignment of nursing personnel for the following day is developed during and immediately after the conference.

Demands on the Professional Nurse

A series of six nursing team conferences was recorded and analyzed by Chao and Willis (9), students of the Division of Nursing Education, Teachers College, Columbia University.

Nine demands were identified in this study.

To identify the patient's nursing problem

The team leader is first of all a listener, for it is through listening that the professional nurse is able to assist the group to develop a whole plan out of the many and varied contributions. As she listens she is able to sift, to relate, to add her own observation, and to evaluate that which is pertinent to the nursing care of the patient. She is then able to guide the group in the identification of the problem and assist them to plan for the nursing care involved. This by no means implies that she does not verbally participate but means rather that the initial emphasis is on providing the team members with an opportunity to explore and evaluate the nursing care they have provided the patients.

To recognize ability and limitations of various team members

The team leader must exercise professional judgment in evaluating the observations, contributions, and suggestions made by other members for the development or evaluation of nursing care. She must also help the team members to recognize their capabilities and limitations in the areas of skill, knowledge, and judgment.

To communicate

The professional nurse must continually be concerned not only with her own ability to communicate but with the ability of the team members as well. It takes two people to communicate—the speaker and the listener. Successful communication in the team depends upon how much understanding the professional nurse may have of the ability and limitations of the other team members. She must be able to recognize when communication barriers exist and what interferes with communication in a group discussion, and she must be prepared to employ approaches which will facilitate communication.

To use scientific information to influence the course of nursing care

This is the expression of the professional status of nursing. It is this ability which makes it possible to plan for comprehensive or individualized nursing care and enables the nonprofessional members of the team to help in planning and evaluating as well as participating in the actual nursing care. Professional knowledge and judgment are reflected in direct proportion to the ability of the professional nurse to recognize any valuable clue in the work, attitude, or thinking of the nonprofessional member, and to identify and apply those scientific principles which would be the most helpful in making use of the worker's contribution.

To generalize from specifics

The leader, in evaluating the contribution of the team members, arranges and presents this information in such a way that it will be useful to the team members at a future date, should a similar situation arise.

To report, interpret, channel, and carry out hospital policies

Policies are necessary guides and as such are subject to interpretation. In team conferences, questions or problems relating to hospital policies are discussed as they apply to particular patients. One policy which frequently comes up for discussion in the conference is that concerning visiting hours.

To teach in conference what is required to help team members fulfill their roles

One of the characteristics of a professional person is the possession of a broad scientific background which may be used in a variety of situations. The nonprofessional person is dependent upon routines or techniques. This difference in background is a basis for the demand for on-the-spot teaching by the professional nurse in the conference. It is important that the professional nurse recognize when teaching is indicated, and whether the teaching will be effective. Detailed teaching is not the responsibility of the team leader in conference.

To plan nursing care cooperatively with other team members

This is the primary over-all purpose of the nursing team conference and as such is an inherent part of all demands made on the professional nurse. The team leader encourages all team members to participate in the planning, and guides the development of the plan on the basis of scientific principles. The planning is always for the individual patient. The nursing care plan is immediate and also long term, and is projected for the patient's return to his home and family.

To bring out "maximum creative potential" of group

The team leader is responsible for creating a working environment which is conducive to the full participation of the member of the nursing team.

It is through the team leader's understanding of, respect for, and acceptance of the members of the nursing team that this environment is fostered. She must be aware of the needs of the members of the group and must assist them to meet these needs. Through this process the team leader assists the other members to identify and to solve problems and thereby to become more competent within the range of their ability. This is directly reflected in their heightened ability to perform more efficiently the actual procedures of patient care.

7. INDIVIDUAL NURSING CARE PLANS

INDIVIDUAL WRITTEN nursing care plans are the guides used by the members of the team. The development of a written plan based upon the individual patient's response to his health problems insures that the patient and his problems will be the basis for assignment, rather than routines or orders. Assignment of members of the nursing team is based upon an evaluation of both the patient's nursing needs and the ability of the personnel to assist him in meeting these needs.

Routine patient care creates hazards. The use of nursing care plans which are developed by the nursing teams eliminates undesirable dependence upon such routine. Assignments are individual, but the written care plan provides a means of communication which safeguards and promotes continuity of nursing care.

Form for Recording Nursing Care Plan

Leino (37) presents the form which is used in the Teaching Demonstration Center. Although this form has been adapted by the nursing service personnel to that particular agency, it is offered as a guide to any hospital planning to develop the team method. (See Exhibit IV, pages 88-89.) Each nursing service should develop a workable form which will meet its own needs.

The form used for recording the nursing care plan is a pair of 5" x 8" file cards. One card presents the patient's identifying data, and information under the headings "Problems" and "Approach" (the plan of the nursing team for assisting the patient in the solution of these problems). On the second card are recorded the objectives of nursing, and treatments and medications administered (delegated by the medical staff as a nursing responsibility).

The cards are filed in a Kardex or visible file—one Kardex for each team—thus facilitating handling and insuring availability.

Developing Nursing Care Plan

The plan is started upon admission of the patient to the ward unit. Identifying data can be copied by a ward clerk and filed immediately in the Kardex. In the initial phase, implications for the nursing care plan are identified by the graduate nurse through her contact with the patient on admission, with the physician, or upon examination of the patient's record. Interviewing the patient upon admission is a professional responsibility and provides a means for the immediate inclusion of the patient in his plan of care. Through this procedure, many factors are identified which have a definite effect upon the adjustment of the nursing care plan to the individual patient. The patient's immediate response to hospitalization, individual needs expressed by him, implications in the medical history—such as impaired hearing or vision—and in the social history serve as illustrations.

The objective of nursing is formulated as soon as the patient's nursing needs are identified. It is specific for the patient and may change, depending on nurse-patient relationship and the response of the patient to this total plan of care.

Following admission of the patient, all members of the nursing team having contact with the patient share in the development of the plan. The regular period for developing and revising nursing care plans is during the nursing team conference. In the process of evaluation of the nursing care provided, problems are identified and an approach is developed for the solution of these problems.

All graduate nurses are responsible for keeping the plan up to date. A change in doctor's orders, conferences with members of the interprofessional health team, or contacts of nursing service personnel with the patient and family often have implications for the nursing care plan. Pertinent information should be entered immediately and shared with the members of the nursing team having contact with the patient.

The nursing care plan, if it is to be functional, must communicate to the nonprofessional as well as the professional members of the nursing team. Simple, concise terminology must be used. The problems identified may be as familiar as "Turning the patient in bed," but the approach for assisting him should be explicit and should include *all* aspects which vary from the routine.

Problems associated with the emotional or physical response of the patient should also be included, as well as implications for nurse-patient relationship. The approach to these problems is based on an understanding of the needs of the individual patient, and on the application of scientific principles to those needs. Confidential information about the patient is not included. Only those problems are identified which affect provision of nursing care or the worker-patient relationship.

The nursing care plan complements the patient's record but in no way replaces it. Nurses' notes are progress reports of the response of the patient to his plan of care.

8. ON-THE-JOB TRAINING PROGRAM FOR THE NURSE'S AIDE

AUXILIARY WORKERS are persons carrying out duties necessary for the support of nursing service, including those duties which involve minor services for patients performed under the direct supervision of professional or practical nurses. Their activities *do not constitute the practice of nursing and therefore there is no reason for them to be licensed.* (48)

In the Teaching Demonstration Hospital a special committee was formed with supervisory, head nurse, and general staff representation, for the purpose of investigating the duties of auxiliary workers authorized by the hospital, and to compare the findings with recommendations made by the New York State Nurses Association. (48)

A list of duties was compiled under the heading, "Responsibilities Which May Be Assumed by the Nurse's Aide." The deciding factors in whether or not an activity should be assigned to an aide were the type of illness of the patient, the response of the patient to his illness, and the anticipated effect of the particular activity. A list headed "Duties of . . . " tends to become accepted as fact, the assumption being that the duties listed are to be performed by the worker under any circumstances. This mistaken assumption may be on the part of the worker himself or of the person responsible for assignment of personnel.

The committee referred the job description to the over-all nursing service staff for evaluation, revision, and approval. The final draft was then referred to hospital administration and approved. It was recognized that it is the responsibility of hospital administration to contact the medical staff or other department heads if a change in policy affects other groups, and that approval of the medical staff is necessary for procedures or routines associated with patient care.

Any printed list or outline should be interpreted if the cooperation of the group is desired, for the rationale gives meaning to the finished product. Presentation of the duties which may be assumed by the nurse's aide requires an interpretation of non-nursing activities—a recommended part of the orientation of all newly employed nursing service personnel.

Non-Nursing Duties

The rationale for differentiating between non-nursing and nursing activities, as accepted by the nursing service staff, is here presented.

Certain activities performed by the nursing staff in the hospital are also performed by the individual or members of the family in the home, in the daily routine of living and maintaining health. The response of the individual to illness and the change in environment from the home to the hospital affect the degree to which the individual or his family can carry out these activities. Examples are bathing, nutrition, and elimination.

The environment of the home may influence the decision as to whether or not to hospitalize, when the sick person is a member of a family group. The mother in the home with small children may of necessity be admitted to the hospital for supervision of health service, whereas the children or husband in the same family situation may be cared for at home. The care of a member of the family requiring bed rest and limitation of activity, primarily, is readily assumed by the wife and mother under the direction of a physician. If she becomes ill under similar circumstances and if her husband is employed, resources within the family may not be adequate for home care of the patient.

The availability of services of the public health nurse is a vital determinant in the care of a patient in his natural environment, the home. The dependence of the individual upon others for service and the resources within the home influence the choice between hospital and home in the evaluation home visit. In the supervision of health services the public health nurse may assume certain aspects of care and delegate other aspects to members of the family. In some situations the individual himself may assume major responsibility except for certain treatments and the over-all supervision which is exercised by the public health nurse. Thus, the availability of public health nursing service in the community influences hospitalization of certain groups of patients.

The well-adjusted individual, capable of dealing with average life situations but temporarily limited physically, can be assisted by a nurse's aide in administering self care if in the home the same service can be provided by a member of the family or a friend. The type and degree of physical disability are recognized as factors in deciding whether or not a nurse's aide can be assigned. Under the circumstances stated, it is assumed that the patient can take on the major responsibility for supervision and direction of the services necessary for his immediate needs.

Frequently a patient will need help with his bath, the ambulatory patient sometimes needing assistance merely in the provision of towels, wash cloth, and soap. A bed patient who is able to bathe himself and to direct the placement of equipment may be assisted by a nurse's aide, who participates only to the extent of washing and rubbing the patient's back and caring for his environment.

Content of Training Program

Preparation of the nurse's aide for active participation as a member of the nursing team is the over-all purpose of the on-the-job training program. Analysis of the relationships involved and of the scope of assignment of activities is the first step. The Teaching Demonstration Center accomplished such analysis by dividing the areas of instruction as follows: (1) responsibility which may be assumed by the nurse's aide, (2) employment of the worker as a member of the nursing service staff of the hospital, (3) the nurse's aide as a member of the nursing team, and (4) relationships of the worker to patients and their families.

Responsibilities which may be assumed by the nurse's aide

Responsibilities approved by the nursing staff and hospital administration in this study were grouped into the following broad categories:
Food service
Housekeeping
Maintenance of supplies
Care of the patient
Transportation and communication
Activities within each category are not specified because the final authority must be individual hospital policy. The types of patients, their nursing needs, the general ability of auxiliary personnel, and resources within the nursing service staff for teaching and supervision are examples of areas to be evaluated in each nursing service situation.

Employment of the worker as a member of the nursing service staff of the hospital

Orientation to environment and personnel
Relationship of worker to other personnel
Personnel policies which affect the worker
Over-all hospital policies and routines
Nursing service policies and routines
The worker as an individual

The nurse's aide as a member of the nursing team

Team relationships
Team functioning
Responsibility to team
Contribution to team

Relationships of worker to patients and their families

Personal hygiene and maintenance of normal body functions
Response of patient and his family to illness
Human relationships in the hospital environment and their effect on
a patient's response to illness and therapy.

The general content of the fourth category was included and developed as a result of evaluation by the nurse's aide group and graduate nurse personnel of the Teaching Demonstration Center of the initial on-the-job-training program. Contact with patients and families in the ward unit and participation as members of the nursing team emphasized the need for this broader concept.

Personal hygiene had first been included in activities concerned with the care of patients. To be meaningful, it must relate also to the worker. If the worker does not practice washing his hands after elimination at home, and does not understand the effect of such neglect upon his own and his family's health, it is useless to expect him to carry out this practice in the hospital environment. Verbal acceptance without understanding does not insure practice.

It is recommended that the discussions of personal hygiene and maintenance of normal body functions center around the needs of the average person rather than those of the patient in the hospital. Discussion of problems of the individuals in the group, or at least problems with which they are familiar, will stimulate interest and personal involvement. Transfer can then be made to the patient in the hospital.

This approach serves two purposes: education of a lay group in health practices, and preparation of this group for patient contact.

Included in this category is an introduction to simple anatomical terms. Since communication is important in worker-to-worker or worker-to-patient relationships, common hospital terminology is discussed. A free discussion clarifies misconceptions.

The demonstration hospital, as has been said, is a cancer hospital, and many stereotypes exist in the lay group regarding this disease process. Observation of the nurse's aide group in the work situation, the type of questions they asked, and the comments they made clearly indicated a need for orientation to cancer. Some of the aides thought cancer was contagious; others that every patient was going to die, therefore treatment was cruel and unnecessary. These are just two of many misconceptions which existed in the group, but they clearly demonstrate the effect they might have in the relationship of the aide to the patient. A sizeable number of the group requested that information about cancer be included in their program.

Another reason for providing the nurse's aide groups with factual information is a discernible assumption of the public that personnel in hospitals have access to general knowledge about matters of health and disease, and therefore can be contacted for information. Observations made in the hospital environment are misconstrued unless the basic elements for understanding are provided. Factual knowledge helps remove the component of mystery, and that which is not mysterious does not incite the false imaginary responses too often accepted by patients and their families.

The personal contacts in the hospital environment are numerous. The role of an individual as a member of a group is magnified by the complexity of the various groups in the hospital. The nurse's aide on a typical patient unit will have contact with professional nurses, practical nurses, aides, patients, families, visitors, doctors, dietary personnel, housekeeping personnel and others. Some of these contacts will be direct, some will be indirect.

Job satisfaction and productivity are dependent upon the individual worker's understanding his relationship to others and upon the development of a functional relationship. Group analysis of problems of interpersonnel relationships experienced by the aides as members of the nursing team or in contact with patients or other personnel develops understanding of human relationships. This process assists the worker to develop an awareness of the effect of emotional responses upon his relationship with others and fosters a better understanding of self.

A successful worker-patient relationship, regardless of the role of the worker, requires an appreciation that changes in behavior may and do occur under the stress and strain of illness and that the relationship can and does influence the response of the patient to his environment.

Method of Teaching

Auxiliary personnel are employed in groups on specified dates. If it is impossible to begin their employment on the day classes are scheduled, they are assigned to simple duties in the central supply room or the operating room. They do not have direct contact with patients until they have had an orientation period.

The on-the-job training program is three weeks in length. (See Figure 4.) The hours, eight to four-thirty, are the scheduled hours of the day tour of duty. During this period, the amount of time spent in instruction decreases as practice, or periods of participation in ward activities, increases.

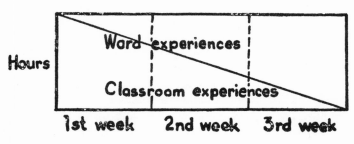

FIGURE 4

After orientation to a specific activity in the classroom, the nurse's aide is given the opportunity to practice under supervision on the ward unit, thereby contributing directly to patient services. The ward participation is increased by the introduction of additional activities, for the practice is cumulative. After a demonstration and discussion of bedmaking in the classroom, the aides continue to practice making empty beds every day. Following an introduction to the serving of diets and the feeding of patients, they participate in this activity as a regular part of their practice period. The classroom experiences are planned around the routine times of ward activities to permit continuity in the practice periods.

One member of the nursing service staff is employed full time for teaching and supervising the auxiliary workers and practical nurses in the orientation period. She also assumes major responsibility for other aspects of the ongoing in-service program for this group.

During the training period the aides are assigned to the instructor. She plans with the head nurses for ward experiences and is responsible for supervision. The aides' names do not appear on the ward time sheets and they are considered additional help at the time they are in the ward for practice. This method has advantages in the response of ward personnel. The general response is that extra help is provided during practice periods rather than that ward personnel are reduced when the group attends class.

The introduction of the nurse's aide to the nursing team precedes orientation to patient services. The instructor assumes the role of team leader for the group during their practice periods. Individual contact with the instructor is available on the wards, and group discussion is provided each day in the classroom. Discussion is centered on observation and activities which are recorded by the aides in their notebooks, and serves as an introduction to participation in the nursing team conference.

Group discussion of personal experiences with patients or with other workers is a technique used to develop observation and communication skills and, thereby, a better understanding of people. The instructor stimulates participation through direct or indirect methods, encouraging the nurse's aides to consider and discuss their various observations and experiences in the ward. The resources within the group are explored by the group members.

The relationship and contributions of the aides to the nursing team and to patient services are thus defined by the group. Examples of key questions which stimulate observation are:

What were the patients doing in the ward? Were all the patients in bed? Were some out of bed? Were they sitting in chairs? Walking about?

Were the patients talking to one another? If some were not, what were they doing? Did the patients talk to other personnel? To you? What was the general conversation?

When you were doing something for a patient, how did he act? What did he say to you? Did he ask questions about his illness, the doctors, nurses, etc.? What were his exact words as you remember them? How did he look when he said this? Did he smile or frown? What did you say?

These questions illustrate simple observations which could be made by the aide and which would contribute to the over-all evaluation of the patient's response and his nursing needs. The assimilation and final evaluation are the responsibility of the professional nurse. but the very presence of others in the patient environment at a time when the professional nurse is not available indicates the desirability of encouraging and directing their observations.

On the other hand, interpretation is not encouraged; rather, the observer is taught to use the patient's own words in reporting conversations with him. He is also encouraged to describe rather than interpret facial or postural expressions, general activity, and deviations from normal physical reactions, such as vomiting, diarrhea, bleeding, and difficulty in breathing.

Availability of the instructor and of the team leader, when assigned to a patient unit, is essential for continuity of care and communication. The discussion period or nursing team conference allows for a cumulation or sharing of the total experiences of the group but does not replace the immediate and direct contact of the nonprofessional personnel with the professional nurse.

It had been noted that one member of the nursing service staff assumes major responsibility for teaching and supervision of the orientation programs of the nonprofessional groups. Additional members of the nursing service and of other departments in the hospital also participate, teaching the care of supplies and equipment by charge nurse of central supply, the preparation of the patient for surgery by the operating room supervisor, the serving of diets by the dietitian, and the setting of personnel policies by the director of nurses or her assistant. Head nurses and general staff nurses rotate in the teaching of selected techniques. This provides for more active participation in the program, with a resultant sharing in development and interest in achievement. The members of the program also benefit from exposure to personnel who are directly concerned with activities which they themselves will perform when they find themselves in an actual work situation.

At times, other personnel participate in the teaching program, leaving the instructor free to observe progress of previous students; to plan individual or group conferences with supervisors, head nurses, team leaders, or former students; to evaluate progress and needs of the group; or to plan for classes.

The methods used in teaching are primarily demonstration and discussion, with a minimal amount of lecture. The lecture method does not stimulate active participation and the span of interest is limited. It is suggested that methods be used which are similar to those employed by the Red Cross in teaching the home nursing courses or by industry in their training programs.

The success of the program and the ability of the nonprofessional personnel to become participating members of the nursing team depend to a large degree upon the skill of the professional nurse in the techniques of communication. Words or concepts which are a part of a professor's accepted pattern of speech rarely have a similar meaning, or even a familiar sound, for a lay group. It has been said that each profession tends to develop its own language.

The ability to interpret or transpose technical words into simple thoughts which will be understandable to those outside the profession is essential for the nurse in her association with lay groups, either patients or workers in the hospital.

It is a relatively new experience for the majority of professional nurses to participate in a teaching program for auxiliary workers. In these teaching programs, intercommunication has been facilitated by the following techniques:

The development of one major theme or concept as one learning experience.

The use of action words to introduce the various steps for a given set of directions. (Refer to sample nursing techniques, Exhibit II, page 84.)

The careful selection and introduction of only key words at the time these words are significant to some action which is being taken, or to some visual symbol.

Use of word symbols which have meaning to the group.

Simple, concise presentations followed by discussions, and re-emphasis or repetition as indicated.

Avoidance of abstract terms.

The use of visual aids.

Continuous observance of the verbal or nonverbal response of the group as a means of evaluation of the level of comprehension.

The maintenance of an environment which encourages free discussion, questioning, and evaluation.

The above list is by no means exhaustive. Only through continued experience and conscious practice in the art of communication can the professional nurse really communicate effectively.

9. ORIENTATION PROGRAM

FOR THE PRACTICAL NURSE

THE OVER-ALL PURPOSE of the orientation program is to evaluate the needs of practical nurses, and to provide learning experiences which will assist them to develop the knowledge, skills, attitudes, and values considered basic to their participation as members of the nursing team. This takes into consideration the needs of all practical nurses, both the trained and the untrained.

Characteristics of Practical Nurses

At the Delafield Hospital a committee was appointed to analyze the preparation and experience of the practical nurses on the staff. Analysis revealed that a majority of the group were graduates of accredited practical nurse schools; that two had been enrolled in three-year hospital schools of nursing and had withdrawn in the third year for reasons of health; and that the remainder were licensed by waiver and had no formal preparation. All were licensed in the state of New York. The ratio of trained to untrained practical nurses changed constantly.

A wide range in the scope and quality of experience existed in both the trained and the untrained group. Curriculum differences in schools for practical nurses and personnel policies of hospitals employing practical nurses were the two primary causes for this variation in the responsibilities which were assigned to the practical nurse. In some situations, practical nurses were assigned activities usually thought to be those of the nurse's aide, the opposite extreme being the situation where the practical nurse was "in charge" of a patient unit without the direct supervision of a professional nurse.

Observations of the adjustment of practical nurses to Delafield Hospital and previous experiences of graduate with practical nurses led to the assumption that in general the preparation and experience of the practical nurse were primarily concerned with routines; that they did not prepare her to adapt previously learned practice or techniques to a new and different situation.

This committee also reviewed the list of duties of practical nurses as set up by the Department of Hospitals of New York City, and this list was then compared with recommendations in *Practical Nursing—An Analysis of the Practical Nurse Occupation with Suggestions for the Organization of Training Programs* (19) and in *Practical Nursing Curriculum* (20). These various recommendations were found to be very similar in content.

The review of this list of duties resulted in a hospital job description which was accepted by the nursing service staff as being a good description of the participation of the practical nurse on the nursing team. In the revised form, a change was made in the job description heading, and the definition of the practical nurse was omitted. (20)

The former heading, "Duties of the Practical Nurse," was changed to "Responsibilities Which May Be Assumed by the Practical Nurse."

The definition of a practical nurse, as accepted by the profession at large and as presented in *The Practical Nursing Curriculum,* is as follows:

A practical nurse is a person trained to care for subacute, convalescent, and chronic patients requiring nursing services at home or in institutions, who works under the direction of a licensed physician or registered professional nurse, and who is prepared to give household assistance when necessary. A practical nurse may be employed by physicians, hospitals, custodial homes, public health agencies, industry, or the lay public. (20)

The foregoing definition was omitted from the newly revised job description because it did not express the philosophy of nursing team assignment. The classification of patients as subacute, convalescent and chronic tends to emphasize the *physical* but neglect the *emotional* response of the patient and his rehabilitative needs.

One sees in the preceding definition an inference that practical nurses are prepared to provide nursing care for patients who require physical care primarily, but that this degree of physical dependence is such that it is possible for the patient to participate in his own care.

In testing the meaning of the definition with representatives of the graduate nurse group it was discovered that the large majority were of the opinion that the degree of physical illness had been the determining factor in the assignment of practical nurses; other components had not been particularly influential.

As a result of this phase of the study, the following new definition for practical nurses is suggested for consideration:

The trained practical nurse is prepared to provide nursing care, under the supervision of a professional nurse, to those patients who primarily require physical care; the degree of dependence for physical care being such that the patient can participate to a degree in carrying out or supervising this care. In assigning responsibilities to the practical nurse as a member of the nursing team, consideration is given to the *selection of the patient* in terms of the total plan of nursing care based on the patient's problems, the *selection of the practical nurse* in terms of ability to perform, and the *adequacy of supervision*.

Development of Program

An orientation program for practical nurses must consider and meet the needs of both the trained and the untrained members of the group. It is one phase of a continuous in-service program.

The ability to perform an act, or to know *how* it should be done, does not imply that the individual knows *what* he is doing or *why*. Skills which are essential in the performance of the personal service of nursing are dependent upon knowledge and judgment. Attitude of the performer toward both herself and the others involved is a strong factor in achieving desirable outcomes. More cooperation will result when the new way seems to offer greater satisfaction to the persons concerned.

Differences in the level of competence of the trained and untrained group are greater than individual differences experienced in a similarly prepared group. This can be seen in any evaluation of performance. Neither the orientation program nor the continuous in-service program is intended to develop a common level of competence within the practical nurse group. Rather, the intent is to assist the individual members of the group to develop to the height of each person's potential, recognizing the limits of an in-service program. The limitations of an in-service program as compared to a program in an accredited practical nurse school must be recognized.

The orientation program which is conducted initially is concerned with the adjustment of the group to the particular hospital situation. It incorporates the learning experiences which are considered to be elementary to the participation of the practical nurse as a member of the nursing team. The wide range of individual differences in both the trained and the untrained group is recognized and dealt with later on through the continuous in-service program. The common areas of activity for practical nurses are those recognized as basic for the nurse's aide also. Although the areas are common, the two groups operate on a different level of endeavor.

Responsibilities which may be assumed by practical nurse

A major difference between the function of the practical nurse and that of the nurse's aide lies in the category of activities concerned with the care of patients. The nursing techniques and routines included can be classified into two groups: (1) those which are considered an activity of nursing or are delegated to nursing, and for which the nursing service staff assumes full responsibility; and (2) those which are considered an activity of the medical, laboratory, or other staffs, and for which the nursing service staff assumes an assisting responsibility.

The job description is used in the orientation of the practical nurse and serves as a guide to the scope of her activities. In her orientation is included a discussion of the basis for assignment of members of the nursing team to patient care. The job description can also serve as a check list of previous experiences. One symbol can be used to check the activities which the individual has previously participated in. A different symbol can be used for graduates of a practical nurse school, to check the activities which she has not participated in but which were included in the teaching program. Analysis of such a check list assists in the development of the orientation program.

Summarization into the following categories serves as an initial step in evaluating the needs of the group.

Experiences common to all members of the group.
Experiences of the major portion of the group.
Experiences of a limited number or none of the group.

These three categories should be examined to identify such activities as differ in method or procedure from the general routines followed in other hospitals. Hospital policies and routines, medical policies and routines, and equipment used are factors which vary in different hospital situations.

A further differentiation can be made between activities which require a general group orientation and those for which the orientation can be done more expeditiously on an individual basis.

Each of the activities on the check list is then examined in terms of the knowledge and judgment considered essential for execution of that specific activity.

As a result of this completed analysis, a differentiation is made between those responsibilities which may be assumed by the total group and those which may be assumed by selected members of the group, the criterion for selection being the preparation and ability of the individual practical nurse. The continuing in-service program should meet the on-going needs of the total group and, through the continuous process of group evaluation, should recognize and provide for individual member differences.

Employment as a member of nursing service staff

This phase of the orientation program for the practical nurse is similar to that suggested in Chapter 8 for the nurse's aide.

The practical nurse as a member of nursing team

The "areas of instruction" (outlined in Chapter 8) concerning nurse's aides are applicable to the practical nurse group also. The extent to which the discussion is carried varies in relation to the role of the practical nurse as a member of the nursing team.

Personal relationships within the nursing team require particular attention. Certain problems can be anticipated in any group situation, but the development of good team relationships is facilitated if the professional nurse fully understands her feelings toward the contribution of the practical nurse to patient care, and that the practical nurse's previous experience will influence her response to new situations. Group exploration and analysis of the members' feelings will help to identify some of the problem areas.

Relationships within a nursing team may be such that they constitute a threat to the security and individual satisfaction of the practical nurse, particularly if she perceives her role as being in a middle position on the nursing team. A strained relationship will result if feelings of pressure are anticipated from above and below. The nurse's aide who is on-the-job trained may be as well prepared as some of the untrained practical nurses. The practical nurse who is licensed only by waiver and who was previously employed as a nurse's aide may be struggling with feelings of ambivalence. In certain patient situations, the assignment of the practical nurse or the nurse's aide may present little apparent difference to the casual observer. Increasing the activities of the nurse's aide may be thought of as encroaching on the prerogatives of the practical nurse.

Also, the practical nurse may perceive the team leader as interfering with or as barrier to communication with the head nurse, the person "in charge." If the practical nurse has previously assumed major responsibility for patient care with relatively little supervision, the direct supervision of the team leader may foster feelings of inadequacy, rather than stimulate personal growth.

These and other forces have been identified as influencing tension areas in the relationship of practical nurses with nurse's aides or graduate nurses. The recognition of potential forces, and the use of the problem-solving method in group discussions of them, facilitate the reduction of such tensions. A good introduction to team relationships is the discussion of feelings concerned with previous incidents which involved interpersonal relationships. This stimulates the development of an environment in which the group members feel free to discuss immediate personal problems.

The process used in discussion will be presented more fully in Chapter 10. Analysis is primarily to explore feelings which have resulted from specific behavior and to discuss, in the group, the possible outcomes of the incidents, were the behavior modified.

The purpose of this method is to assist the practical nurse to develop an appreciation of the effect of behavior on relationships with others, and to be aware of and accept the importance of individual responsibility for the effective functioning of the nursing team. It follows that job satisfaction and productivity of the nursing team are directly proportionate to the quality of patient care provided by the nursing team. As the group becomes secure in the process, the influence of personal conflict upon patient services is emphasized, for a disturbed worker transfers the disturbance to the patient.

Relationships to patients and their families

Again, the general outline of points to be emphasized in the program is comparable to that developed for the nurse's aide. The differences in the relationships of the practical nurse will depend upon her previous experience and the responsibilities she will assume as a member of the nursing team.

This phase of the program emphasizes the physical and personal relationships of the worker to the patient. The nature of the activities and of the practical nurse's contact with the patients, as compared with the non-nursing activities and contacts of the nurse's aide, requires on the part of the practical nurse, a general understanding of the patient's health problems and also of the contribution which may be expected of her to the total plan of nursing care for the patient.

A concept of optimum health is necessary to an understanding of the factors affecting health and the response of the individual to these factors. Maintenance of health and the prevention of diseases are introduced in a discussion of personal hygiene and normal body functions. The term personal hygiene is familiar to the nonprofessional group and is used in the discussion to indicate those health habits desirable in daily living. Specific examples are used to illustrate individual differences caused by age, sex, culture, and race.

The character of the discussions is determined by a variety of needs, it being assumed that individuals in the group will have different degrees of understanding. A discussion which is not instructor-dominated will activate the individual members who have particular understandings and will provide a means for group evaluation of their needs. Points which require particular emphasis are identified through this process. The lecture method is avoided, since it inevitably leads tc repetition of experiences within the group which are better presented individually. Repetition is productive only if the members of the group have the experience of sharing and contributing to the development of the discussion.

In the process of the discussion, the instructor summarizes the group's contribution as each major point is developed, supplements points requiring additional information, and introduces new or unfamiliar information. The emphasis is placed on health as a prerogative of all people and as a concern of the practical nurse in her personal life, as well as in her association with patients in the hospital.

Since the demonstration hospital (Delafield) is selective, admitting patients for diagnosis, treatment, and research in cancer or allied diseases only, an introduction to cancer as a major health problem was included in the orientation program. Provision should be made, in the in-service program of the practical nurse who is employed in a general or special hospital, for an orientation to the major health problem encountered. The participation of the practical nurse in nursing care presupposes an understanding of basic essentials affecting the patient's physical response to illness.

The information concerning major health problems which is presented to the general public through special educational services, radio, television, daily press, and other media emphasizes that the hospital, as a health agency, should assume responsibility for seeing to it that the personnel are at least as well informed as the general public.

Regardless of the major health problem of the patient, or the plan of medical care, certain principles of general nursing are considered to be applicable to all patients. Special needs or problems will modify the individual patient's plan of nursing care. A review of the common elements of nursing as they affect the contribution of the practical nurse to patient care is helpful as a means for introducing nursing techniques and routines to the group in association with patient problems.

The modification of a routine to a special need and the nature of the problem which created the special need influence the assignment of the practical nurse.

Following an orientation to the common elements of nursing and to the routines which affect the nursing care of all patients, there should be an orientation to the modifying of patient routines in the different clinical services. For example, in the genitourinary service the following points are emphasized:

Measuring intake and output. (Reasons for and importance of accurate measurement; the method of procedure; observations of deviations from normal color, amount, bleeding, pain, and so forth.)

Care of the patient with an indwelling catheter. (Purpose of urinary drainage; equipment and procedures used; arrangement of tubing to prevent tension or pressure when the patient is in bed, in a chair, or ambulatory; observations of drainage.)

Care of the patient with a perineal prostatectomy. (Measures used to control the patient's desire to defecate; purpose and meaning of "no rectal treatments"; position of suture line and the effect rectal thermometers and rubber rings have in the healing process; purpose and procedure in the administration of heat to the perineum; general routine for personal care. Pajama pants irritate the suture line and should not be worn.)

Each service presents modifications in the routine as a result of the nature of the surgical or medical therapy. Additional examples are:

Modifications in the control of the environment for the patient with a communicable disease or receiving radioactive isotopes.

Meeting the nutritional and emotional needs of the patient with a gastrostomy.

Physical and emotional response of the patient with a colostomy.

Posture, position, and exercise as it affects the patient with an orthopedic problem.

The effect upon respiration, communication, and emotional response of a patient with a tracheostomy.

The examples cited illustrate modifications in common elements of nurse-patient relationship; ability of the patient to communicate with others; posture, position, and exercise; control of the environment; maintenance of normal body functions (urinary elimination, bowel elimination, respiration, and digestion); and the emotional problems inherent in each of the situations presented.

Human relationships in the hospital environment and their effect on a patient's response to illness and therapy are an integral part of the discussion of every situation involving the worker and the patient.

There is always danger that in the routine of hospital life, concern with the acquiring of skill in the many nursing techniques will overshadow the patient. Too often emphasis is put upon skills in working with equipment and secondary consideration is given to the skill of working with people.

The term "human relationships" rather than "interpersonal relationships" is used to describe the interaction of people. "Human" is a familiar term in the vocabulary of the group whereas "interpersonal" is an abstract and unfamiliar term. "Personal" to the group usually means "self"; the prefix "inter" frequently only adds confusion. An unfamiliar symbol can be a serious block to understanding a concept.

A discussion of human relationships isolated from an actual situation is only an observation and can easily turn into a discussion of the other fellow. Too often a patient is classed as difficult without any examination of the factors in the environment which might have contributed to the feelings behind the criticized behavior. Stereotypes do exist as to acceptable behavior, and the patient who does not conform may be classified in accordance with stereotypes.

Participation as a member of the nursing team provides a continuing opportunity for developing an understanding of the process of human relationships. In the orientation program, problems of practical nurse-patient relationships experienced by members of the group in providing nursing care are discussed in relation to the total experience.

Method of Teaching

The orientation program for practical nurses in the demonstration hospital is two weeks in length and includes active participation in the ward units. Approximately three and one-half hours are devoted to group orientation and the remainder of the time to individual orientation through participation in ward activities. The practical nurse is assigned to a nursing team following the first day of orientation to the hospital, personnel, personnel policies, and nursing team organization.

Effective functioning as a member of the nursing team is the result of a gradual growth process. A verbal introduction or the mere presence of an individual within the organizational framework of the nursing team does not insure active participation as a team member. The orientation to nursing team functioning is provided through participation in ward activities and through associated group discussions. As has been said previously, the individual becomes a functioning team member, or the collected individuals become a team, only when the satisfactions derived from working as a unit outweigh the satisfactions of working alone.

A full-time instructor assumes responsibility for the orientation programs of both the nurse's aides and the practical nurses. Since the practical nurse is immediately assigned to a ward unit, the head nurse and the team leader also assume major responsibility, with other graduate nurses or department heads participating. The program is planned to permit participation on the ward during the peak of the work load and participation in selected experiences. During the period the practical nurse is on the ward unit, the instructor plans with the head nurse and with the team leader for group experiences, such as a demonstration of a particular nursing technique, or participation in the nursing team conference. She also assists in the supervision of the group.

During the process of supervision the instructor, who is free from ward responsibility, is able to assist in the adaptation of routines or techniques. Because of her contact with the practical nurse in the patient environment the instructor is better able to assist the group members evaluate their needs. Familiarity with patient problems and with the environment is essential because the entire program is experienced-centered.

The team leader, head nurse, instructor, and the newly employed practical nurse share in continuous evaluation. The assignments are adjusted until a specific activity in the orientation program is completed or until the practical nurse demonstrates satisfactory understanding and skill through actual practice under the supervision of team leader, head nurse, or instructor.

In certain instances the program assumes the nature of on-the-job training; in other instances, that of a refresher course. The problem of preparing trained and untrained members simultaneously influences the program.

The discussion of methods of teaching and communication which were suggested for the auxiliary personnel also applies to the practical nurse group. Every opportunity should be provided for personal involvement of the individual, either in discussion or in practical experience. The attainment of skills in working with people, in manual dexterity, in communication, and in other necessary areas is best accomplished through practice in an environment conducive to personal growth.

10. IN-SERVICE PROGRAMS FOR THE GRADUATE NURSE

THE PURPOSE OF an in-service program is improvement of nursing service. Provisions for stimulating the growth and development of members of the staff are directly reflected in the increased competence of that staff. An in-service program for professional nurses must be planned for a particular hospital in terms of the needs of its graduate nurse group, and in terms of their function in that particular agency. The in-service program should be continuous and should evolve as the needs of the personnel change.

Expansion of health services and increased demands for the participation of the professional nurse in these services require nurses who are capable of quickly becoming oriented and functioning members of the health team. This implies a professional nurse who is capable of defining her role in any situation; one who has developed the ability to assess the complex situation and reduce it to its component parts, thereby identifying the abilities, skills, or knowledge she requires to function in the situation. She can also recognize and locate resources necessary to the solution of any problem.

The preparation of the staff nurse is accomplished by an in-service program in which she develops her ability to function as a *member of the health team* and as *leader* of the nursing team. It is assumed that the in-service program will of necessity be complementary as well as supplementary to her basic preparation.

As has been stated previously, the needs of any specific group of graduate nurses will determine the nature of the in-service program. A group evaluation of problems is indicated in developing any in-service program.

In the course of the study it became evident that there were two distinct aspects of the in-service program in the Teaching Demonstration Center. One aspect—the unplanned—developed as the need arose in particular situations involving a group or individuals; the other aspect—planned—was developed by the staff for a unit, for a group of units concerned with common problems, or for the total staff.

No attempt will be made to outline a total in-service program in this written report. Instead, methods used to assist the graduate nurse group with specific problems, as these problems relate to their functions as team leaders or team members, will be presented as examples or guides.

Introduction to Nursing Team Organization and Functioning

Provision must be made, by any agency planning to institute this program, to contact all graduate nurse personnel presently in their employ, as well as those who will be employed at future dates. This includes the day, afternoon, and night staff.

One effective method of contacting the currently employed staff has been to have representatives of the three shifts of duty participate in the initial discussion, following which the supervisors have conducted a continuation of the discussion with the remainder of the staff at a convenient time.

In the Teaching Demonstration Center all graduate nurses, regardless of their position, have an orientation period on the day shift before being assigned to afternoon or night duty. It is during this orientation period that the nursing team organization and functioning are explained.

Role of Team Leader

During the course of the study it became evident that problems associated with the functioning of the graduate nurse as team leader relate directly to specific activities. The emphasis in the in-service program centered around problem areas rather than around the role of the team leader, even though it is a complex one. This emphasis permitted clarification of the role of the professional nurse as a practitioner and also the identification of the knowledge, skills, abilities, and values inherent in team leadership. It is a building-upon, rather than a complete reorientation to, the role of the professional nurse.

Identification or Diagnosis of Nursing Problem

Since the Teaching Demonstration Center was a specialized hospital for the treatment of cancer and allied diseases, and since the majority of nurses have not had basic training or experience in this highly specialized service, it was anticipated that they would have need for it. Certain problems which arose, associated with the development of nursing care plans and with participation in the nursing team conference, were directly related to a need for general knowledge of cancer as a health problem and to an understanding of the plan of medical therapy as practiced by the medical staff of this hospital. Insecurity of the professional nurse in the clinical area was reflected in her relationship, as team leader, to the nonprofessional members. In repeated instances, a general evasion was observed if an interpretation or explanation relative to cancer was requested.

The problems experienced in the development of nursing care plans were explored by the graduate nurses, and the inability to identfy nursing problems was usually associated with the need for information in the area of nursing care of the patient with a diagnosis of cancer. Therefore, a general course in cancer nursing was offered to provide the nursing staff with such a background. At the request of the staff, this course was content-centered.

Concurrently with the class in cancer nursing, a problem-centered nursing conference was held. The purpose of this conference was to assist the nursing group in the identification of problems and in the application of scientific principles to planning and to the providing of nursing care. Patients were selected for discussion by the participants, and their problems were identified and classified into two groups: (1) those common to any nursing situation; (2) those peculiar to the patient whose major health problem was cancer. This was an attempt to lessen the emphasis on cancer, and to center the development of the nursing care plan around the problems of the patient.

The group discussion in the problem-centered conference included an orientation to the patient and his family, the health problems of the patient, the patient's and family's adjustment to the health problems, the medical care plan, the nursing problems identified, the present and projected plan of nursing care, and the rationale for the plan. The rationale was based upon the physical, mental, emotional, spiritual, and social principles relating to the individual problems of the patient and his family.

The supervisory staff of Delafield Hospital and the instructional staff of Teachers College acted as resource people in this discussion. As a result of the discussion, a nursing care plan was developed for a patient or a group of patients.

Immediate concern with the medical diagnosis and plan of therapy often negates other important aspects of care. Components of care which are taken for granted by a graduate nurse are often those which are the most important for the nonprofessional personnel to be aware of in providing nursing care. Anticipation is a safeguard in planning for nursing care. It is not possible to assume or take for granted that everyone knows a certain component is important. There is relatively little common know-how or know-why in the situation which includes nurse's aides, practical nurses, and graduate nurses.

Another method used to assist the graduate nurse in the identification of nursing problems was provided through conferences with the medical staff. Changes or new developments in medical practice and research directly affect nursing practice. The joint conference provided an opportunity for identification of the implications for nursing and the development of a plan by the nursing staff to provide for the nursing aspects of care. Medical-nursing planning conferences should be provided for on a continuing basis, to insure individualized nursing care.

Relationship of Team Leader to Team Members

Relationships within the organizational framework of the nursing team directly affect the functioning of the various members as a team; organization alone does not insure team functioning.

The graduate nurse as team leader must be sensitive to problems of interpersonal relationships or worker-to-worker relationships, and the effect these problems have on the worker. Tension can be avoided in the work situation if the team leader is aware of those conditions which create tension and conflict. The process involved in directing and supervising the work of others is based upon a knowledge of the art of human relationships.

During the course of the study, in the Teaching Demonstration Center, the graduate nurses, head nurses, and team leaders met in groups to explore incidents which they felt had created tension, conflict, hostility, and so on, either in their own response or in the observed response of other members of the nursing team. The person involved described the incident, which included the setting (whether head nurse unit, patient unit, or some other place); the persons involved; verbal interchange; nonverbal or behavioral communication; and the feelings associated with the experience, either felt or observed. The group then analyzed the incident to determine the factors which might have influenced this particular response. Following the identification of problems which appeared to create blocks, the group explored possible approaches which might have fostered a productive worker-to-worker relationship instead.

This method serves to stimulate awareness that the words one selects, the manner, the tone of voice, the facial expression, and the posture of the body affect the response of others.

Leadership in Nursing Team Conference

Several methods were used to introduce the graduate nurse to her role of leader of the nursing team conference.

If the nursing service is in the process of initiating nursing teams, a role-playing demonstration serves as an introduction to the conference, as well as to the roles of the team leader and the head nurse. A graduate nurse skilled in group leadership should function in the roles of team leader and head nurse.

This demonstration method has also been effective in analyzing the problems encountered in the nursing team conferences and in further assisting the group to develop skills in leading a group discussion. In a role-playing demonstration, graduate nurses can assume the roles of the nonprofessional members of the nursing team and can present problems which are most frequently observed in the nursing team conference. Following the role-playing demonstration, the part played by the leader can be analyzed for its effectiveness or ineffectiveness: as to whether or not it accomplished the purpose of the conference and whether or not the techniques of leadership were demonstrated.

New employees "sit in" on several nursing team conferences as a part of their orientation program. The supervisor who is responsible for the orientation discusses the purposes of the nursing team conference and the role of the team leader in it prior to the demonstration. Following the conference, the supervisor and the group or the individual being oriented analyze it as to accomplishment of purpose and effectiveness of the team leadership role.

Continuation of this phase of orientation is assumed by the head nurse. When assigned to a ward unit, the graduate staff nurse observes a series of conferences before assuming the leadership role. When she does assume team leadership, the head nurse and the beginning team leader plan for a brief evaluation period following the actual team conference. If the head nurse is unfamiliar with the conference procedure, the supervisor assuming over-all responsibility for assistance in the development of a nursing service or a nursing team assumes this function.

Nursing Team Assignments

Nursing team assignments are dependent upon the preparation of the individual worker and the emotional and physical response of the patient to his health problem. The range of activities is clearly defined for each group of workers, but assignment requires individual evaluation of the patient's nursing needs and evaluation of the ability of the individual members of the team to assist the patient in meeting these needs. All graduate nurses are oriented to the scope of activities which may be assumed by the nurse's aide or the practical nurse.

The instructor of the nonprofessional group works closely with the graduate nurse staff in planning the in-service program for the non-professional members of the nursing team. Opportunities are provided for their observation and participation in this program. Continuous and final evaluation, at the end of the initial on-the-job training program for the nurse's aides and the orientation program for the practical nurses, are shared with the supervisors, head nurses, and team leaders. Strengths and weaknesses of the individuals are identified to be used as guides for the planning of assignments and for their implica-tion of the potential needs of the team members for guidance and supervision.

The head nurse assists the new team leader in developing the details of the assignment plan and provides continuous supervision of the development and implementation of the plan.

Nursing Service Organization

Participation of the nursing service staff in the formation of depart-mental policies and procedures and in the solution of problems is provided by organization of the nursing service department. The head nurses and supervisors have a scheduled meeting once a week, the general staff nurses meet on a "needs" basis. Other committees are formulated for specific purposes, in terms of jobs to be done. Oppor-tunities are provided for all members of the nursing service staff to participate in committee work.

A natural outgrowth of participation in committee work which is directed at the improvement of nursing service is the development of skills in problem-solving.

Continuous Evaluation of Nursing Team Functioning

One of the most productive experiences of this study has been the wholehearted participation of the entire nursing service staff in the evaluation of nursing team functioning. Meetings are scheduled at frequent intervals, at the request of the staff, to evaluate progress. Problems associated with the development of nursing teams are iden-tified and plans are revised or developed in view of those problems. In-service needs of personnel are identified and planned for at these meetings.

11. NURSING TECHNIQUES APPLIED TO THE NURSING TEAM

THOSE STUDENTS who are registered in the Division of Nursing Education, Teachers College, for the course "Relationships and Team Functions in Nursing" participate in the study and design of a nursing technique (or procedure) for the use of the nursing team. To do so, the students form groups which function as nursing techniques committees. The Teaching Demonstration Center is used as the control situation and the techniques are designed for that agency. The nursing service, medical, or laboratory staffs of the cooperating hospital; instructional staff of the Division of Nursing Education, Teachers College; and personnel from other agencies cooperate as the need is indicated.

Nursing techniques are classified into two groups: those which are considered an activity of nursing, or are delegated to nursing and for which the nursing staff assume full responsibility; and those which are considered an activity of the medical, laboratory, or other staffs, for which the nursing staff assumes an *assisting* function.

Hospital policies which relate to the functions of nursing personnel are guides in considering which group or groups should be involved in the performance of specific procedures.

Exploration by the nursing service staff, in conjunction with the medical staff, indicated a need for the preparation of all personnel in certain skills and understandings associated with nursing techniques which might at times be emergency in nature. These techniques were usually considered to be a professional responsibility. Examples are: suction of the tracheostomy tube, and clamping of the chest tube attached to chest drainage. (See Exhibits II and III.) Although the graduate nurse is assigned the patients needing such care, in an emergency everyone should be aware of the procedure, so as to facilitate immediate action. This includes the family, and housekeeping as well as nursing personnel. Immediate suction is imperative if the tracheostomy tube becomes plugged, and immediate clamping of the chest tube is equally imperative if the connections to the drainage bottles becomes dislodged. The person who is present and who recognizes the patient's need calls for a professional nurse or a physician but remains with the patient to administer emergency care. If the housekeeping personnel are aware of the need to use caution in moving a drainage bottle, a safeguard is instituted.

The above examples fully illustrate the need for developing a format for nursing techniques which will be understandable to all concerned.

The developing of nursing techniques is a responsibility of the professional nurse, for although the end product may be merely a routine, or directions for procedure, that end product is the result of scientific investigation and of the application of scientific principles.

The writing of directions is a skill which requires special emphasis. Steps of procedure must be expressed simply and concisely if the directions are to be clearly understood and quickly followed by anyone concerned—professional nurse, student, practical nurse, or nurse's aide. The majority of forms for written directions of nursing procedures fail to follow basic rules of communication. The style in which the directions are presented, and the symbols used, should communicate clearly to all who will need to read them.

The ease with which directions are read is in direct relation to the length of the sentences and the complexity of the words. When developing a format acceptable to the Teaching Demonstration Center (see Exhibit II), the "command" type of sentence was decided upon. Sentences are begun with verbs—action words.

Word symbols used are those which have common meaning for all concerned. Drawings are used freely, because visual symbols tend to make unnecessary the complex or abstract descriptions. That which can be visualized is more readily understood.

The organization of material is another important factor in communication. The equipment or articles to be used are listed in the left column so that the assessment of necessary equipment can be quickly made by reading down that column. In addition, these listings appear in the column directly opposite the directions for the use of that particular piece of equipment. Thus, in reading across the page, a relation will be seen between the equipment, the directions, and the reasons for carrying out the procedure. However, the organization also permits the identification of each of these items separately. Each step can thus be clearly identified for the reader and quickly checked later, should the need arise.

It is recognized in developing a format for a nursing technique that its primary purpose is to direct. If the nursing technique is unfamiliar to a group of workers or students and is introduced in an in-service or teaching program it will be supplemented through the process of teaching.

It is assumed that if all three groups are concerned in carrying out a technique, one written nursing technique could be developed. If the various groups of nursing service personnel are to carry out a certain nursing technique, the directions for carrying out that technique should logically, and functionally be the same.

12.   ORGANIZATION OF A HOSPITAL NURSING SERVICE ON A TEAM BASIS

THE PLAN OF organization suggested here is the result of: (1) the initial study of the organization of a ward unit on a team basis by Leino; (2) the intensive study and experimentation by members of the nursing service of the Francis Delafield Hospital and of the project staff of the Division of Nursing Education of Teachers College in the organization of the hospital nursing service on a nursing team basis; (3) the experience of the writer through consultation service to other hospitals, with the resulting contribution of the nursing service personnel of these hospitals; and (4) the continued interest and contribution of students in the Division of Nursing Education through their participation in field experience at the Teaching Demonstration Hospital, the Francis Delafield Hospital.

Reorientation of Nursing Staff

Change is a gradual process and initiation of change should be evolutionary, not revolutionary, in nature. The term "reorientation" is used to point up the fact that change from a familiar to a new and strange system of operation is merely a change of one's position, or of the relationships within the environment. Nursing service personnel already employed in hospitals have been oriented to their role in nursing service through educational experiences, in-service programs, or work experience. The purpose of all nursing services is the same, regardless of the organizational pattern. A shift from traditional practice to participation as a member of the nursing team does not change the purpose in any way—it changes only the methods by which those purposes are achieved.

The familiar system of providing patient care may have seemed a comfortable one wherein the members of the staff concerned themselves only with their immediate assignments and their primary responsibility to immediate "superiors." On the other hand, the relationships within the team and the responsibilities inherent in these relationships may constitute a threat to the security of the individual if changes are perceived as losses of individuality or of status.

This uneasiness has been identified in the study through verbal communication and through observation of communication expressed in behavior.

For example, the graduate nurse may feel threatened and tension may result if, in her opinion, the practical nurse, as a team member, is infringing on the prerogatives of the graduate nurse. The practical nurse, in turn, may fear that pressure from the graduate nurse will limit her contribution. She may also feel her position threatened by the nurse's aide who is prepared on the job. This tension is particularly noticeable in the practical nurse who has had little direct supervision and who has, in previous employment, assumed primary responsibility for nursing care. The nurse's aide may resent the additional responsibility inherent in being a team member if she has previously been satisfied just to carry out repetitious tasks. These are a few of the responses which may be anticipated, depending upon the previous experience of the group.

The manner in which any proposal for change is first introduced is vital in securing the interest and participation of the group. If the nursing service personnel are not already familiar with the nursing team functioning, an introduction of the philosophy and mode of operation is indicated, prior to any decision for such change. It is necessary to success that those who will be directly concerned with the change be a part of the group who make the decision.

Several methods have been employed for the introduction of nursing team functioning to nursing service personnel. Two which have been successful are: the use of a resource person from outside the agency; and the preparation of a member of the staff through observation visits, work conferences, and other means. If the resource person is not a member of the staff, she should be familiar with the immediate nursing service situation and the problems of which the group are already aware. The introduction should be in terms applicable to the particular agency. Building upon the familiar is constructive, and also economical in time and energy. The emphasis is upon reorientation in the introduction as well as throughout the process of change.

Assessment of Problems

The nursing team is not a cure-all. If problems exist in the nursing service department, or in its relationship to other departments, they will continue to exist if no conscious attempt is made to identify their source or to provide a workable solution.

A positive approach is a group exploration of problems which interfere with direct service to patients. In the Teaching Demonstration Center, for instance, a number of small group conferences were held to decide upon the quality of nursing care which the nursing team desired to provide, to identify any factors which might prevent the attainment of such a standard. Nurse's aides, practical nurses, and graduate nurses participated from the day, afternoon, and night staff. These conferences were held at times convenient to the different shifts in order to provide an opportunity for each group to identify the problems peculiar to it. If the problem was one of nursing service, it was placed in the agenda of a regular staff meeting. If it was interdepartmental it was referred by the director of nurses to the hospital administrator for departmental consideration.

In several other hospitals an Institute was planned as part of an in-service program. Following an introduction of the philosophy and method of functioning of the nursing team, areas of interest were selected for investigation by small groups. The process was one of problem-solving. For example, one group selected for discussion the nurse's aide as a member of the nursing team. In order to anticipate problems which might arise from participation of the nurse's aide in the nursing team, they explored problems being currently experienced by the group. They then attempted to identify the root of the problem. Was it orientation, selection of personnel, or what? Next, the group examined current practice in an attempt to decide whether or not the services of the nurse's aide were being fully and effectively utilized. Job specifications of the nurse's aide as determined by hospital policy, the New York nursing law as it defined the function of the auxiliary worker, the in-service program provided, the employment policies, and so on were explored.

Following this phase of the group discussion, the participants identified changes which they thought were desirable in hospital policy, in the in-service program, and so on to enable the nurse's aide to function effectively as a member of the nursing team. As a result, the various small groups made definite recommendations to all participating in the Institute.

The Institutes were planned on a two-day basis, with time arranged for the nursing service personnel to participate one of the two days. A general evening meeting on the second day provided an opportunity for the two groups to meet. As a result of this a committee was selected, by the combined groups, to develop a blueprint of procedure for the organization of the nursing service on a team basis. The plan was to be based upon the recommendations of the small groups.

In the process of developing the Teaching Demonstration Center on a nursing team basis, the staff recognized the need for group meetings. Two three-day work conferences were planned. Scheduling of time on duty provided for participation of the graduate nurse staff at one or the other of the conferences. The purpose of the conferences was to provide an opportunity for the graduate nurses to meet to evaluate progress, to identify problems hindering the development of the nursing service, and to plan for further development of the nursing service on a team basis.

The participants were purposely selected to provide for representation at each work conference from the day, afternoon, and night staff as well as from the staff nurse, head nurse, and supervisory personnel. The conferences were held in May, four months after the first group of patients were admitted, and the number of graduates involved was therefore relatively small.

The hospital administrator, medical staff, and department heads met with the groups as the need arose. During this period policies and routines were established, nursing techniques examined for revision, and an orientation program was developed for graduate nurses. A major portion of the time was devoted to the clarification of the roles of the team leader, head nurse, and supervisor and to the nursing needs of patients with cancer as a health problem.

Reorientation of Hospital Staff

The various departments of a hospital are interdependent in their provision of services for patients. These services must be coordinated, as must also the activities of the personnel involved. Change in one department may affect its relationship to others. The nursing team, functioning in the patient unit, is in working proximity to the activities of most other departments.

When the decision to change to nursing team organization has been accepted by the nursing service department, a reorientation of other departments is indicated, as is a redefinition of the relationships of the nursing department to other departments. This does not imply a *change* in relationships, but rather a *clarification*.

In several instances during the course of this study, the hospital administrator provided for a meeting of department heads where the director of nursing service presented the reasons for change and explained the purpose of nursing team organization and functioning. A discussion period gave opportunity for further clarification. Department heads assumed responsibility for reorientating other staff members.

In the Teaching Demonstration Center additional conferences were planned with individual department heads and with the nursing service staff. At these conferences the department heads interpreted the functions of the department. After the introduction, a group discussion clarified the relationship of the nursing service to specific departments.

Assessment of Personnel Resources

In the Teaching Demonstration Center, and in other hospitals cooperating either directly or indirectly in the study, the nursing service staff on a ward unit was kept constant. If a unit was organizing on a team basis, personnel were not added at the sacrifice of other units, for the major purpose of the study was not only to improve the quality of nursing care but to do it with the available personnel.

Assessment of the number, kind, preparation, and ratio of professional to nonprofessional personnel on a given ward unit is essential in determining possibilities of team grouping and functioning.

Determining Composition of Teams

The number of teams is necessarily limited by the number of graduates available. The team leader is always a graduate nurse. If on a ward unit there are two graduate nurses other than the head nurse, one team is indicated. With a five-day work week, each of the three graduates is off duty two days. One graduate functions as team leader and the second graduate relieves her for two days, relieves the head nurse for two days, and is off duty for two days. This plan allows for at least two graduate nurses to be on duty each day.

Relief for team members is planned within the team. If two practical nurses are members of one team, they relieve each other for days off. It has been found that planning days off one month in advance allows for individual and group planning and for a satisfactory distribution of time.

If stability of team composition is to be maintained, the number and ratio of personnel should be such that days off are provided for.

It has not been possible as yet to study the most economical and effective ratio of aides, practical nurses, and graduate nurses in the provision of nursing care to a group of patients. Criteria for measuring the quality of nursing care are essential, and a study to set up such criteria is in process at the present time. When it is decided what quality is desirable, then it will be possible to decide the kinds and number of personnel required for a team.

At this phase of the study, certain factors in the demands made on the nursing staff of the various wards have been identified as influencing the composition and number of nursing teams which are required to provide nursing care on a particular ward unit. These factors are:

1. The general plan of medical therapy.

2. The scope of responsibility delegated to the nursing staff, or assumed by the nursing staff as their contribution to the total medical care plan.

3. The extent of physical care required by the patient—complete bed rest, bed, chair, ambulant, and the like.

4. The nature and complexity of the emotional problems of the patient. (The patient with cancer may display intense emotional stress.)

5. The rehabilitative needs of the patient and the teaching needs associated with his physical and emotional response to his health problem.

6. The scope of responsibility which the nurse's aide and practical nurse can assume as defined by hospital policy.

7. The length of hospitalization of the patient.

8. The responsibility of the nursing service staff for assistance with medical research.

9. The responsibility of the nursing service staff for participation in teaching programs for student nurses, medical students, and so forth. (Orientation of medical students to a ward unit is not identified in general as participation in the teaching program, but the demands are extensive in many instances observed.)

10. The physical arrangement and size of the ward unit and the proximity of patient units to service units. Grouping of patients allows for group teaching and supervision.

11. The number and kinds of personnel other than nurses who have contact with patients on a ward unit, using the medical staff as an example—(Do the patients have private physicians? If so, how many different doctors on an average are concerned? Does the hospital supply medical service? If so, how many are involved—attendants, residents, interns, medical students?)

12. The quality and preparation of nursing service personnel for their functions associated with the provision of and quality of the in-service program.

13. The relationship of the nursing service department to other departments in the hospital and the participation of the nursing service staff in policy development, etc.

These thirteen factors have been identified as directly influencing the quality and/or quantity of direct contact of nursing service personnel with patients and, therefore, as having a direct relationship to the composition of nursing teams, as well as to the number of nursing teams on a given patient unit. This list is by no means exhaustive.

Development of a Plan for Action

Following the acceptance, by the nursing service staff, of the fact that a change to nursing team organization and functioning is desirable, it is recommended that an over-all plan be developed for the initiation of such nursing teams. A plan is essential, but it should be subject to modification at any time.

Provision is made in the plan for an evaluation of the over-all nursing service so as to determine which changes are desirable. Such evaluation should precede the actual initiation of nursing teams in a selected unit. This step in planning conserves energy and time in later development of the nursing team organization and functioning in the patient unit.

After the initial evaluation comes the second part of the plan, which is concerned with the actual procedure for initiating nursing teams.

Clarification of the role of the various members of the nursing team into job specifications for the nurse's aide, practical nurse, graduate nurse, team leader, and head nurse serves as a common basis of communication. The members of the nursing team are then familiar with their role and their relationship to other members of the team. The need for clearly defined and written job specifications is emphasized because of the general confusion which has been observed in several situations when there was only an oral interpretation of responsibility. Interpretations varied. Team leaders and head nurses on different patient units in the same hospital showed wide differences in their understanding of the respective responsibility of team members.

Putting the Plan into Action

As a result of the study of the organization of a nursing service on a team basis, it is recommended that one member of the nursing service staff be assigned the over-all responsibility for coordination of those activities which are associated with the initiation of nursing teams. The person selected should function in a supervisory relationship to the head nurses of the various units and should be available for on-the-spot problem conferences, as the need arises. The functions of this person are defined by the over-all planning group and are presented to the nursing staff for consideration and approval. Communication between the various patient units is provided by the appointment of this person. Thus, the loss of service through avoidable trial and error on the part of the various head nurses is minimized.

It is suggested that a test period be conducted in one patient unit at first to allow for modification and adaptation of the principles of nursing team organization and functioning. The test unit will provide an opportunity for experimentation without interfering with the stability of the entire nursing service.

The primary factor in selecting the test unit is that the personnel involved be interested and willing to participate. It is recommended that provision be made in the over-all plan for such selection. This unit should be a representative one, and the staff should have been given the opportunity to volunteer as a test group.

During the trial period, plans are made for communication among the entire nursing staff. Opportunity is provided for progress reports and evaluation. The length of the trial period will vary.

Following the development of the test unit, plans are made to organize other units on a team basis. Preparation of personnel for the change has usually been facilitated by the use of the initial unit as a means of orientation for the head nurses and for team leaders of other units. Both the head nurse and the team leaders of the next unit to be organized spend some time in the already functioning unit. As more units begin to function, more opportunities are available.

The importance of providing an in-service program cannot be overemphasized. Personnel on the ward unit are responsible for nursing care, and any demands on them to train other workers subtracts from the time they can devote to the patient. It is economical to provide orientation or training of personnel within an organized in-service program. The head nurse or team leader cannot be expected to train the nonprofessional workers. This point is stressed here because it has been observed that in many hospitals there is no provision made for on-the-job training programs, and because nonprofessional personnel are frequently assigned immediately to a ward unit, in which case the personnel of the unit must assume the responsibility for training or teaching this group. Such assignment can only result in a dilution of nursing service and the ineffective training of personnel, thereby increasing the incident of hazard in the patient environment.

It must be remembered that change is a gradual process and improvement of the quality of nursing care through successful team functioning is accomplished only through the participation of all involved.

BIBLIOGRAPHY

1. AMERICAN HOSPITAL ASSOCIATION AND NATIONAL LEAGUE OF NURSING EDUCATION. *Hospital Nursing Service Manual.* New York, NLNE, 1950, p. 99.
2. AMERICAN NURSES' ASSOCIATION. *1951 Facts About Nursing.* New York, American Nurses' Association.
3. ARNSTEIN, MARGARET G. "Our Nursing Needs." *57th Annual Report of NLNE,* 57:314, 1951.
4. BARRETT, MARY V. "An In-Service Educational Program for Nurses." *American Journal of Nursing,* 51:388, September 1951.
5. BENNE, KENNETH D. AND MUNTYAN, BOZIDAR. *Human Relations in Curriculum Change.* New York, Dryden Press, 1951, p. 363.
6. BERENGARTEN, SIDNEY. "When Nurses Interview Patients." *American Journal of Nursing,* 50:131, January 1950.
7. BERENGARTEN, SIDNEY. "The Significance of Interpersonal Relationships." *American Journal of Nursing,* 52:1219, October 1952.
8. BROWN, ESTHER LUCILLE. "Studies in Interpersonal Relationships in the Therapeutic Setting." *Public Health Nursing,* 43:360-363, July 1951.
9. CHAO, GLORIA AND WILLIS, LUCY. "A Study of Demands Made on Professional and Practical Nurses in the Planning Conference of the Nursing Team." Unpublished student study, Division of Nursing Education, Teachers College, Columbia University, 1952.
10. COCH, L. "Overcoming Resistance to Change." *Human Relations,* 1:512, August 1948.
11. COFFEY, HUBERT S. "Role-Playing in Exploring Relationships." *Public Health Nursing,* 42:267, May 1950.
12. COLUMBIA UNIVERSITY, TEACHERS COLLEGE, DIVISION OF NURSING EDUCATION. *Regional Planning for Nursing and Nursing Education.* New York, Teachers College, Columbia University, 1950, p. 69.
13. COMMITTEE ON FUNCTION OF NURSING. *A Program for the Nursing Profession.* New York, The Macmillan Company, 1948, p 108.
14. COMMISSION ON HOSPITAL CARE. *Hospital Care in the United States.* New York, Commonwealth Fund, 1947, p. 631.
15. COMMITTEE REPORT. "Criteria for the Assignment of the Nursing Aide." *American Journal of Nursing,* 49:311, May 1949.
16. COOLEY, CAROL H. *Social Aspects of Illness.* Philadelphia, W. B. Saunders, 1951, p. 305.
17. DEMING, DOROTHY. *The Practical Nurse.* New York, Commonwealth Fund, 1947, p. 370.
18. EMERSON, LYNN A. *How to Prepare Training Manuals.* New York, Delmar Publishers, 1952, p. 356.
19. FEDERAL SECURITY AGENCY, VOCATIONAL EDUCATION DIVISION,

OFFICE OF EDUCATION. *Practical Nursing—An Analysis of the Practical Nurse Occupation with Suggestions for the Organization of Training Programs.* Washington, D.C., U. S. Government Printing Office, 1947, p. 134.

20. FEDERAL SECURITY AGENCY, VOCATIONAL EDUCATION DIVISION, OFFICE OF EDUCATION. *Practical Nursing Curriculum.* Washington, D. C., U. S. Government Printing Office, 1950, p. 144.

21. GARRETT, ANNETTE. *Interviewing. Its Principles and Methods.* New York, Family Service Association of America, 1942, p. 123.

22. GERMAIN, LUCY D. "Continuing In-Service Education." *American Journal of Nursing,* 51:670, November 1951.

23. GINSBURG, ETHEL. *Public Health Is People.* New York, Commonwealth Fund, 1950, p. 241.

24. GILBERT, RUTH. *The Public Health Nurse and Her Patient.* Cambridge, Massachusetts, Harvard University Press, 1951, p. 335.

25. HERROLD, KENNETH F. "Conference Planning and Action Through Use of Group Process." *Public Health Nursing,* 42:199, April 1950.

26. HESTAD, HELEN E. "Hospitals Without Walls." *Public Health Nursing,* 43:447, August 1951.

27. HILDEBRAND, EDITH A. "Listening Is Part of the Job." *Public Health Nursing,* 43:436, August 1951.

28. HOWARD, LOIS M. *"How to Make the Best of Auxiliary Personnel." Modern Hospital,* 76:57, January 1951.

29. JOINT COMMITTEE ON PRACTICAL NURSES AND AUXILIARY WORKERS IN NURSING SERVICES. *Nursing Aides and Other Auxiliary Workers in Nursing Services.* New York, American Nurses Association, 1951.

30. JOINT COMMITTEE ON PRACTICAL NURSES AND AUXILIARY WORKERS IN NURSING SERVICES. *Practical Nurses in Nursing Services.* New York, American Nurses Association, 1951, p. 52.

31. KELLEY, EARL C. *The Workshop Way of Learning.* New York, Harper & Brothers, 1951, p. 169.

32. KITCHELL, MYRTLE E. "Analyzing and Developing Nursing Procedures." *American Journal of Nursing,* 51:174-181, March 1951.

33. LEE, IRVING J. *"How to Talk with People."* New York, Harper & Brothers, 1952, p. 176.

34. LEIGHBODY, GERALD B. *Methods of Teaching Industrial Subjects.* New York, Delmar Publishers, 1946, p. 178.

35. LEINO, AMELIA. "Organizing the Nursing Team." *American Journal of Nursing,* 51:665, November 1951.

36. LEINO, AMELIA. "A Study of Team-Organization of Nursing Personnel." Unpublished Study, Division of Nursing Education, Teachers College, Columbia University, 1950.

37. LEINO, AMELIA. "Planning Patient-Centered Care." *American Journal of Nursing,* 52:324, March 1952.

38. LESNIK, MILTON J. AND ANDERSON, BERNICE E. *Legal Aspects of Nursing.* Philadelphia, J. B. Lippincott Co., 1947, p. 352.

39. LORENZ, MILDRED. "A Progress Report on Nurses' Assistants. *American Journal of Nursing,* 51:304, May 1951.

40. MAGNUSSEN, ANN. "The Teaching Procedure Used in Red Cross Home Nursing." *Public Health Nursing,* 44:21, January 1952

41. MCMANUS, R. LOUISE. "Improving Nursing Through Action Research.' *57th Annual Report of NLNE,* 57:387, 1951.

42. MCMANUS, R. LOUISE. *The Effect of Experience on Nursing Achievement.* New York, Bureau of Publications, Teachers College, Columbia University, 1949, p. 64.

43. MONTAG, MILDRED L. *Education of Nursing Technicians.* New York, G. P. Putnam's Sons, 1951, p. 146.

44. NAHM, HELEN. "Satisfaction with Nursing." *Journal of Applied Psychology,* 32:335, August 1948.

45. NATIONAL HEALTH ASSEMBLY. *America's Health: A Report to the Nation.* New York, Harper & Brothers, 1949, p. 395.

46. NATIONAL LEAGUE OF NURSING EDUCATION, DEPARTMENT OF SERVICE TO SCHOOLS OF NURSING. *Joint Nursing Curriculum Conference:* Curriculum Bulletin No. 2. New York, NLNE, 1951, p. 57.

47. NATIONAL LEAGUE OF NURSING EDUCATION, DEPARTMENT OF SERVICE TO SCHOOLS OF NURSING. *Nursing Organization Curriculum Conference:* Curriculum Bulletin No. 1. New York, NLNE, 1950, p. 112.

48. NEW YORK STATE NURSES ASSOCIATION. *Examples of Non-Nursing Duties for Auxiliary Workers in Nursing Service.* New York, NYSNA, 1949, p. 11.

49. PEPLAU, HILDEGARDE. *Interpersonal Relations in Nursing.* New York, G. P. Putnam's Sons, 1951, p. 330.

50. PEPLAU, HILDEGARDE. "Understanding Ourselves." *57th Annual Report of NLNE,* 57:242, 1951.

51. PETRY, LUCILLE. "Setting Our Sights." *57th Annual Report of NLNE,* 57:322, 1951.

52. PHILIPS, ELIZABETH C. "The Practical Nurse Is on Her Way to a Place on the Nursing Team." *Modern Hospital,* 75:83, September 1950.

53. PIGORS, PAUL AND MYERS, CHARLES A. *Personnel Administration.* New York, McGraw Hill Book Company, Inc., 1951, p. 614.

54. RICHARDSON, HENRY B. *Patients Have Families.* New York, Commonwealth Fund, 1945, p. 408.

55. ROGERS, CARL. *Client Centered Therapy.* Houghton Mifflin Company, New York, 1951, p. 560.

56. SEHL, KATHERINE. "Administrative Training for Nurses." *Hospitals,* 26:70, June, 1952.

57. SEYFFER, CHARLOTTE. "Principles of Supervision and Administration." *American Journal of Nursing,* 51:257, April 1951.

58. SHARP, GEORGE. *Curriculum Development as Re-education of the Teacher.* New York, Bureau of Publications, Teachers College, Columbia University, 1951, p. 132.

59. SIMMONS, LEON. "The Manipulation of Human Resources in Nursing Care." *American Journal of Nursing,* 51:452, July 1951.

60. TROY, CRESCENTICA J. "Let's Start with the Patient." *American Journal of Nursing,* 51:699, December 1951.

61. VIGLIONE, AMY E. "Training Programs for Practical Nurses." *American Journal of Nursing,* 51:297, May 1951.

62. WHEELER, DOROTHY V.   "We Need General Practitioners in Nursing."
    American Journal of Nursing, 51:462, July 1951.
63. WILLIAMS, JANETTE SPURRIER.   "My Orientation to a New Job."
    American Journal of Nursing, 51:42, January 1951.
64. WOLF, LULU K.   "The Nurse as a Person."   *American Journal of Nursing*, 51:176, March 1951.

EXHIBITS

EXHIBIT I

SAMPLE NURSING TEAM ASSIGNMENT

AN ASSIGNMENT for one member of each of the groups is described. This in no way represents the complete assignment for each member of the group or for a typical nursing team. It is intended to show the relationships of assignments and the differentiations of functions.

TEAM LEADER: Miss Jones

TEAM MEMBERS: Mrs. Smith, Miss White, Miss Green

MISS JONES
Patients

Mrs. K.: Complete care

Miss H.: Preparation for surgery at 10 A.M.

Miss C.: Teach self-administration of insulin and test urine

Special Assignments
New admissions
Medications for team

MISS WHITE (PN)
Patients

Mrs. K.: Assist with bath

Mrs. D.: Bed bath (assist)
S. S. enema
Special back care as patient is incontinent

Mrs. A.: Bed bath
Up in chair half an hour
S. S. enema at 10 A.M.

Mrs. E.: Bed bath
Perineal flush after bedpan
Heat light to perineum
To X ray at 11 A.M.

MISS GREEN (NA)
Patients

Miss Y.: Assist with bed bath
Up in chair half an hour
Make bed when patient is up

Mrs. C.: Patient bathes self
Make bed when patient is up

Mrs. A.: Make bed when patient is up
In chair for half an hour

Mrs. B.: Assist with tub bath
Special care to feet and back
Make bed when up
Measure output
Patient to use bedpan

Special Assignments
Clean all bedside stands for patients assigned to team

EXHIBIT II

TRACHEOSTOMY CARE

Definition

TRACHEOSTOMY consists of an incision into the trachea and the insertion of a double cannula through which the patient breathes.

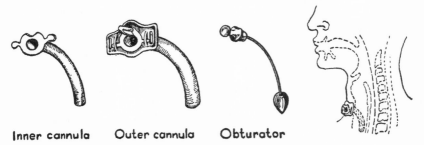

Inner cannula   Outer cannula   Obturator

Things to Be Kept at Bedside

1. Extra sterile tracheostomy double cannula
2. Suction equipment
   Wall suction
   Gauge
   Drainage bottle
   Rubber tubing
   Glass connecting tube
   Whistle tip catheter
3. Small pillowcase
4. Container with clean water
5. Container with obturator, brush, and dilator
6. Emesis basin
7. Tissues
8. Magic slate and pencil (for communication by patient)
9. Mirror (for teaching purposes)

Important Precautions

1. Inner cannulae are *not* interchangeable.
2. If outer cannula should come out and extra one cannot be inserted at once, hold incision in neck open with dilator until doctor arrives, to enable patient to breathe.

3. Silver is soft, handle with care. *Do not drop!*
4. If cannula is cleaned by agent other than water (i.e. hydrogen peroxide or sodium bicarbonate) to remove stubborn mucus, be sure it is rinsed *thoroughly*. Use of other agent should not be necessary if cannula is cleaned often enough.
5. Good oral hygiene (mouth care) is important. Do not neglect.
6. Teach patient to care for himself as soon as possible.
7. Apron over cannula opening may be kept moist to prevent dryness in the trachea, or may be omitted entirely, as the doctor wishes.

Procedure for Tracheostomy Care

PURPOSE: To keep airway passage clean and unobstructed for the patient with a tracheostomy.

ARTICLES NEEDED	STEPS	WHAT TO DO	REASONS
	Prepare patient	Explain what you plan to do	To put patient at ease
Container of water Suction equipment Whistle tip catheter (in small pillowcase attached to side of bed when not in use)	Test equipment	Put catheter tip in water Listen for sucking sound Watch for flow of water into drainage bottle	To be sure equipment is working
	Encourage patient to cough	Put patient in sitting position Hold outer cannula against neck	To bring secretions up To make patient feel secure
	Suction immediately	Pinch catheter Insert 4-5" into inner cannula (unless ordered otherwise)	To prevent waste of oxygen To prevent sticking of catheter to side of cannula To prevent injury and remove mucus plugs below cannula
		Rotate catheter Withdraw quickly	To clean all sides To let patient take a breath
		Put catheter tip in water Repeat suction process until airway passage is clear	To clear equipment of mucus

ARTICLES NEEDED	STEPS	WHAT TO DO	REASONS
	Remove inner cannula	Hold outer cannula against neck Unlock inner cannula by turning flag up Take out inner cannula	To prevent cannula from coming out
Brush Running water	Clean inner cannula	Place under running water Clean inside with brush Rinse well, shake off excessive water	To clean easily and prevent use of other agents, do this as often as needed
Placement of trachea tube	Replace inner cannula	Suction outer cannula if needed Insert inner cannula Lock by turning flag down	To keep cannula in place
4 x 4* gauze square cut to center	Check tape and dressing	Make sure tape is tied securely with 2–3 square knots, a little to midline back of neck Change dressing if soiled	To prevent cannula from coming out To protect skin
4 x 4* gauze square tape	Make apron	Open gauze square, fold halfway over tape	
	Apply apron	Place gauze square over cannula and tie tape at side of neck	To keep out foreign bodies

* *Not Cotton Filled*

Prepared May 1952

Betty-May Bancroft   Adria del Rosario
June Clermont   Stella Koziol
          Eva M. Wohlauer

EXHIBIT III

UNDERWATER CHEST SUCTION

PURPOSE: To drain the pleural cavity without permitting the entrance of air which would cause lung collapse.

EQUIPMENT	DIRECTIONS	PRINCIPLES
Drainage Bottle— *Sterile*		
1 large bottle	Fill bottle to approxi-	To maintain negative
1 two-hole rubber stopper	mately 1½ inches with sterile water	pressure and receive drainage
1 long right-angle glass tube		
1 short right-angle glass tube		
1 long rubber tube		
1 glass connector		
Safety Bottle— *Unsterile*		
1 large bottle	Fill bottle ¾ full with	Safety device to regulate
2 short right-angle glass tubes	tap water	the pressure to which patient is subjected
1 long glass tube		Length of air vent tube
1 long rubber tube		determines the amount
1 short rubber tube		of negative pressure.
1 three-hole rubber stopper	Assemble and set up ar-	Each cm. below sur- face of the water
2 bottle racks	ticles as shown in dia-	equals 1 cm. of nega-
1 large safety pin	gram	tive pressure.
Source of suction		

Procedure

1. Patient returns from O. R. with catheter from chest clamped off.
2. Connect catheter to drainage bottle.
3. Connect tube from safety bottle to wall suction and turn on suction.
4. Remove clamp from catheter.
5. Pin drainage tube to bed, leaving ample tubing to allow patient movement.
6. Clamp off tube nearest chest when emptying drainage bottle.

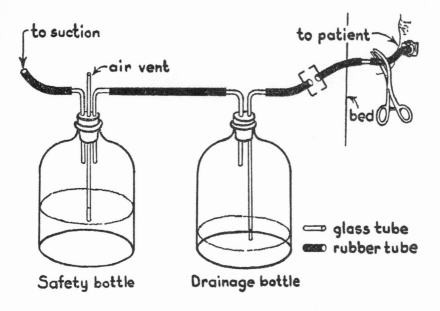

Safety bottle   Drainage bottle

glass tube
rubber tube

Caution

1. Always keep bottles below level of patient, and tubes and air vent under water.
2. Clamp off tube nearest chest immediately for emergency.
3. Fluctuation of fluid in glass tube should occur with each respiration. This indicates that the connection with the pleural cavity is patent.
4. Air vent in safety bottle should be at point of bubbling to see that apparatus is working at desired pressure.

Note

Use Y glass connector if patient returns with two chest catheters.

Prepared May 14, 1952

Annie Gamble   Louisa Jekel
Betty Ito   Mazie Kaku

EXHIBIT IV

NURSING CARE PLAN

PATIENT'S NAME: John C.

HOSP. NO.: 54/23   SERVICE: G.U.

OBJECTIVES OF NURSING: To recognize the patient's need for independence and to assist the family to face the patient and his family in meeting these needs. To assist the family to face the inevitability of death, and to plan with the family and public health nurse for a productive experience for the remainder of patient's life span

MEDICINES	TREATMENTS
Demerol 100 mgm PRN	Nasal oxygen
Penicillin 300,000 U. Q4H	Attach catheter to
Streptomycin 0.5 gm	straight drainage.
Prostigmine 1:4000 Q4H	Attach chest catheter
Mineral oil 15 cc BID	to underwater drain-
Vit. B. Complex 6 cc BID	age. Do not tamper
Thiamine chloride 100 mgm	with bottle or tubing.
with ginger ale BID (P.O.)	If bubbles are not
Na. luminal 120 mgm	seen in water from
with ginger ale PRN	tube, clamp off
for restlessness.	catheter. Notify
	Doctor immediately.
	Fowler's position when
	fully reacted.

88

NURSING CARE PLAN

GENERAL NURSING	PROBLEMS	APPROACH
DIET: Soft regular as tol.	Wants to be treated like a man."	Do not try to fool patient. Do not talk down, or baby him.
T.P.R.: Q 4 H (rectal)		
FLUIDS: Small amts. water freely		
BATH: Bed	Skin very tender due to many infusions & malnutrition.	Handle gently with smooth, slow motions.
ACTIVITY: Bed, up in chair, ambulant	Lack of appetite. "Stomach always feels full."	Try 6 small feedings daily. Encourage to take milk or fruit juice.
SPECIAL NEEDS	Lies in bed staring into space. General lack of interest in self.	Family to bring in fish aquarium. Show interest.
Development & provision of new interests. See priest & family re former interests.	Cannot see reason for getting out of bed. "Feels too weak."	Include patient in planning for time out of bed.
Family think patient would be happier at home with friends available.	Life expectancy. To return home. Mother & Father depressed & anxious	Contact and plan with Public Health Nurse for home care.

DATE ADM.: 11-3-51   DATE DISCH.:

OPERATIONS: Biopsy, retro-peritoneal mass, right nephrectomy.

DIAGNOSIS: Cancer of kidney

AGE	NATIONALITY	RELIGION				FAMILY	
15	American	Catholic.	S	M	W	D	Mother, father & younger brother

ROOM	BED	NAME	HOSP. NO.	DOCTOR
512	2	John C.	54123	Smith